THE
PALM OIL
MIRACLE

DR. BRUCE FIFE

Piccadilly Books, Ltd.
Colorado Springs, CO

Grateful acknowledgment is given to Daabon Organic USA for the photos used on pages 4, 13, 23, and 137 and the Malaysian Palm Oil Council for the photos on pages 12, 44, 53, 72, and the photos of the palm trees on the cover.

Piccadilly Books, Ltd.
P.O. Box 25203
Colorado Springs, CO 80936, USA
info@piccadillybooks.com
www.piccadillybooks.com

Library of Congress Cataloging-in-Publication Data
Fife, Bruce, 1952-
   The palm oil miracle / by Bruce Fife.
      p. cm.
   Includes bibliographical references and index.
   ISBN-13: 978-0-941599-65-8
   1. Palm oil--Health aspects--Popular works. 2. Trans fatty acids--
Health aspects--Popular works. 3. Essential fatty acids in human
nutrition. I. Title.
   QP752.T63F54 2007
   613.2'84--dc22
                                          2007000074
Printed in USA

Contents

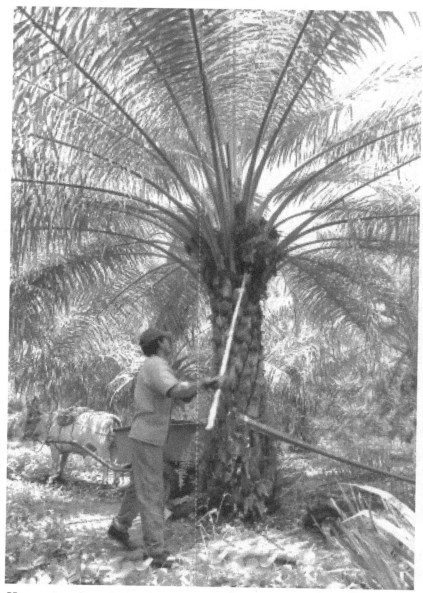

Harvesting fruit from the oil palm (Elaesis guineensis).

Chapter 1

An Exceptionally Good Fat

Asmah, age 9, like many children living on the island of Sumatra in Indonesia suffers from malnutrition. Earthquakes, flooding, and tsunamis that devastated the area in recent years have made life in his village difficult. When the sun goes down, Asmah is afraid to step outside his home. At night he is in total darkness. Asmah suffers from night blindness caused by a vitamin A deficiency. Without sufficient light he is totally blind. If caught outside when night falls, he could wander aimlessly—a terrifying experience to a child.

Night blindness is so common in many areas of Indonesia that the people have a special name for it: *buta ayan*, which means "chicken eyes." The name comes from the fact that chickens are unable to see at night. Mothers seeing their children wandering about, stumbling, and falling because they can't see is heartbreaking. When the sun goes down, many children just sit on the ground like chickens throughout the night waiting for sunlight to reappear.

Like other children in the village, Asmah has difficulty in school. Vitamin A deficiency has affected not only his ability to see but to learn as well. Other symptoms include anemia, growth retardation, painful joints, weakened teeth, hyperkeratosis (hard white lumps on the skin), and low immunity resulting in frequent illness.

Vitamin A deficiency is the major cause of childhood blindness in the world, destroying the vision of a quarter of a million preschool children each year in Asia alone. It is estimated that more than 5 million children worldwide are affected by vitamin A deficiency.

In order to stop this disease, governments have initiated nutritional programs with varying degrees of success. One of the difficulties in treating this disease is that food sources of vitamin A are generally expensive, and vitamins are beyond the financial means of many. Unrefined or red palm oil is now being used with great success in reversing this devastating disease. The oil is relatively inexpensive and can even be produced locally in many of the affected areas. It is used in cooking, replacing other oils with essentially no extra expense.

How does red palm oil correct vitamin A deficiency? Red palm oil contains a rich source of beta-carotene which the body can convert into vitamin A. As a result, Asmah and other children like him are given a second chance at life. Blindness is stopped, growth rates increase, bones and teeth become strong, illness is less frequent, and learning improves. All these benefits occur without changing the diet in any appreciable way except to add red palm oil.

The benefits of using red palm oil extend beyond just supplying a source of vitamin A. It also improves the body's ability to absorb other

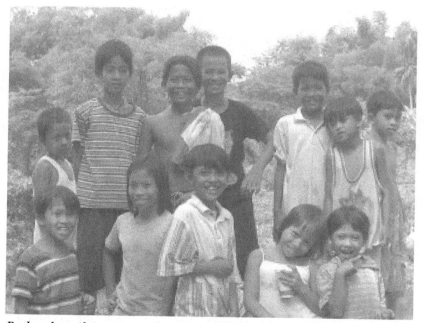

Red palm oil is saving the lives of children who often suffer from nutritional deficiencies.

fat soluble nutrients such as vitamins D, E, and K and improves the body's ability to absorb important minerals such as calcium and magnesium, all of which are essential for normal growth and development and overall good health. Because of the success of pilot programs like the one that saved Asmah, palm oil is being used in many countries around the world to fight malnutrition.

Even in countries where vitamin A deficiency is not considered a major health problem, like in the United States, palm oil is finding a place as part of nutritionally improved dietary programs in schools. Schools seeking to provide children healthier meals are cutting back on sweets, sodas, and foods fried in hydrogenated vegetable oils. Schools are providing children with more fresh fruit and healthier beverages, and are cooking in trans fat-free palm oil. The biggest problem with the hydrogenated vegetable oils used in restaurants and schools is that they contain harmful trans fatty acids. With medical authorities now encouraging us to avoid hydrogenated vegetable oils, food manufacturers and schools are looking for healthier alternatives. Palm oil provides a perfect solution.

In the wake of an increased awareness over child obesity and diabetes, school districts are retooling lunch programs, hoping to boost nutrition while meeting tight budgets. Troy School District in Michigan, for example, has made the switch from hydrogenated oils to palm oil. "Our school lunch program is a leader in ensuring our students develop healthy lifestyles," says Superintendent Janet H. Jopke. It does not have any of the negative features found in other oils such as artificial colors, preservatives, trans fatty acids, or cholesterol. In addition, it provides many nutrients such as vitamins A, E, K, and CoQ10.

French fries are among the most popular lunch items. Cooked in palm oil, they are now more healthful then they used to be. "We always try to give kids what they want in the healthiest way we can," says Jennifer Haglund, a cook at Larson Middle school. "Fries are a big thing. We offer other stuff, but they want those fries."

As knowledge of the health aspects of palm oil become more widely known, it is being used more frequently in place of other vegetable oils and animal fats, particularly as an alternative to health destroying hydrogenated fats and shortenings.

While it makes sense to replace hydrogenated oils with healthier alternatives, some people may ask: but why choose palm oil? The answer is that palm oil is a very healthy oil, which provides superior cooking and baking qualities compared to most other oils.

The health aspects of palm oil have been extensively studied over the past couple of decades. Consequently, palm oil is emerging as one of the premier oils—superior to most of the fats and oils currently used in our diet. Some of the benefits associated with palm oil reported in recent studies include:

- Helps protect against heart disease
- Improves blood circulation
- Helps protect against many forms of cancer, including breast cancer
- Improves blood sugar control in diabetics
- Improves nutrient absorption and vitamin and mineral status
- Aids in the prevention and treatment of malnutrition
- Is a heat stable cooking oil
- Contains no trans fatty acids or cholesterol
- Supports healthy lung function
- Helps strengthen bones and teeth
- Supports healthy immune system function
- Supports eye health
- Protects the liver
- Helps protect against mental deterioration, including Alzheimer's disease
- Provides a rich, natural source of health protecting antioxidants
- Is the richest dietary source of vitamin E and beta-carotene
- Has the highest natural source of health promoting tocotrienols
- Helps stabilize cells and tissues
- Protects against destructive action of lipid peroxidation
- Helps protect against premature aging

At one time palm oil was criticized as being unhealthy because of its high saturated fat content. It contains as much saturated fat as it does unsaturated fat. Consequently, palm oil was lumped together with other saturated fats by the media and many health care professionals as contributing to heart disease. We now know that palm oil does not contribute to heart disease and should be considered as one of the "good" fats. Unfortunately, many people are still misinformed and

8

continue to criticize it. This has created a great deal of confusion and prejudice against palm oil.

The primary purpose of this book is to educate the reader about the true character of palm oil and encourage its use in place of other, less healthy fats. As you will discover, palm oil, and especially red palm oil, is an exceptionally good fat that is superior in many ways to most other dietary fats.

What the Experts Are Saying About Palm Oil

The following quotations are from medical professionals and researchers who have spent years studying the health aspects of palm oil and its individual components.

"We have that negative view of palm oil in the United States—a perspective I have been trying to change for many years! New studies support the fact that palm oil should indeed have a place in a prudent diet, contradicting a myth that is peculiar only to this country…My friends in the Asian Pacific Rim eat high levels of palm oil and have a very low incidence of breast cancer. Anecdotal, to be sure, but now understood and confirmed by so many reputable studies."
Betty Kamen, PhD.

"A number of controlled human studies in Europe, the United States, and Asia, in addition to animal studies, have confirmed that there is no significant rise in serum total cholesterol when palm oil is used as an alternative to other fats in the habitual diet (providing most of the dietary fat)."
Khalid A. Madani, M.P.H., D.Sc.

"The results of recent research on the effects on blood cholesterol of palm oil (or its liquid fractions like palm olein) agree that the substitution of palm fruit oil for the usual fats in the diet does not result in elevation of blood cholesterol."
Gene A. Spiller, Ph.D, CNS
The Trans Fats Dilemma and Natural Palm Oil

"The benefits of palm oil to health include reduction in risk of arterial thrombosis and atherosclerosis, inhibition of endogenous

9

cholesterol biosynthesis, platelet aggregation, and reduction in blood pressure."

D. O. Edem
Plant Foods for Human Nutrition 2002;57:319-341

"Palm oil is endowed with a good mixture of natural antioxidants and together with its balanced composition of the different classes of fatty acids, makes it a safe, stable, and versatile edible oil with many positive health attributes."

N. Chandrasekharan
Medical Journal of Malaysia 1999;54:408-427

"Owing to its high content of phytonutrients with antioxidant properties, the possibility exists that palm fruit offers some health advantages by reducing lipid oxidation, oxidative stress and free radical damage. Accordingly, use of palm fruit or its phytonutrient-rich fractions, particularly water-soluble antioxidants, may confer some protection against a number of disorders or diseases including cardiovascular disease, cancers, cataracts and macular degeneration, cognitive impairment, and Alzheimer's disease."

Ray Sahelian, MD

"Numerous studies have confirmed the nutritional value of palm oil...Palm oil in balanced diets generally reduced blood cholesterol, low-density lipoprotein (LDL) cholesterol, and triglycerides while raising the high-density lipoprotein (HDL) cholesterol. Improved lipoprotein(a) and apo-A levels were also demonstrated from palm oil diets."

A. S. Ong and S. H. Goh
Food and Nutrition Bulletin 2002;23:11-22

"Dietary supplementation of tocotrienols [in palm oil] may provide significant health benefits in lowering the risk of breast cancer in women."

P. W. Sylvester and S. J. Shah
Frontiers in Bioscience 2005;10:699-709

"Tocotrienols [from palm oil] are one of the most potent anticancer agents of all natural compounds."

Y. Yano, *International Journal of Cancer* 2005;115:839-846

Chapter 2

The Trans Fat Attack

A TRADITIONAL FAT

Palm oil comes from the fruit of the oil palm (*Elaesis guineensis*). It is believed that the oil palm originated in tropical Africa where it was used as far back as 5000 years ago. Archeologists in Egypt have found palm oil residue in earthenware jars in tombs dating back to 3000 BC. Its discovery in Egypt indicates it was a valuable commodity used in trade because the oil palm does not grow in that area.

The oil palm eventually migrated from tropical Africa to South America and Southeast Asia. Beginning in the 16th century, African slave ships coming to Brazil brought seeds with them. It is believed that the slaves were fed a mixture of palm oil and flour during their ocean voyage. Some of the seeds were either discarded or planted in the new land. The warm, moist climate of Brazil provided an ideal environment for the oil palm to flourish.

In the 1840s oil palm was introduced as an ornamental plant in the Dutch West Indies (Indonesia). From there it spread to much of Southeast Asia. Most of the commercially produced palm oil today comes from Southeast Asia. The top nine palm oil producing countries in order of production are: Malaysia, Indonesia, Nigeria, Ivory Coast, Colombia, Thailand, Papua New Guinea, and Ecuador. Malaysia is the world leader in palm oil production and produces more than all the other countries of the world combined. Malaysia and Indonesia together account for 80 percent of the world's production. Palm oil has recently surpassed soybean oil as the most widely used oil in the world.

11

The oil palm is a perennial tree that produces fruit year-round. On well–farmed plantations, its oil yield surpasses that of all other vegetable oil plants, yielding about three times the oil of coconuts and well over ten times that of soybeans per acre.

Palm fruit can be harvested three years after planting. The tree has an economic life of about 25 years. The fruit is about the size of a small plum and grows in large bunches weighing 20-50 pounds (10-25 kg). A tree produces 12 bunches per year, with 1,000-3,000 fruits per bunch. One bunch of fruit is harvested about every month, so production continues year round. Each fruit consists of a hard kernel (seed) inside of a thin hard shell which is surrounded by a fleshy husk (mesocarp). Palm oil is extracted from the mesocarp.

Natural palm oil is an integral part of a healthy tropical diet in Africa and Southeast Asia, just as olive oil is in the Mediterranean region. In West Africa, palm oil is still generally consumed in a crude state. The oil is obtained readily from the flesh surrounding the seed by cooking, mashing, and pressing. The oil has been extracted in this manner for generations and locally every family makes their own. The oil is then used in traditional foods, where it contributes its characteristic color and flavor to the dishes.

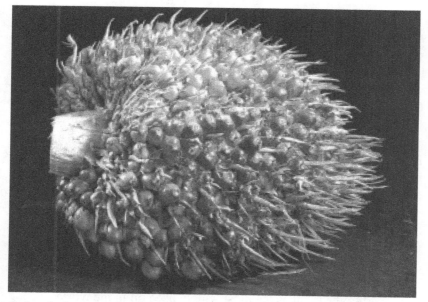

Palm fruit grows in bunchs containing as many as 3000 fruitlets.

12

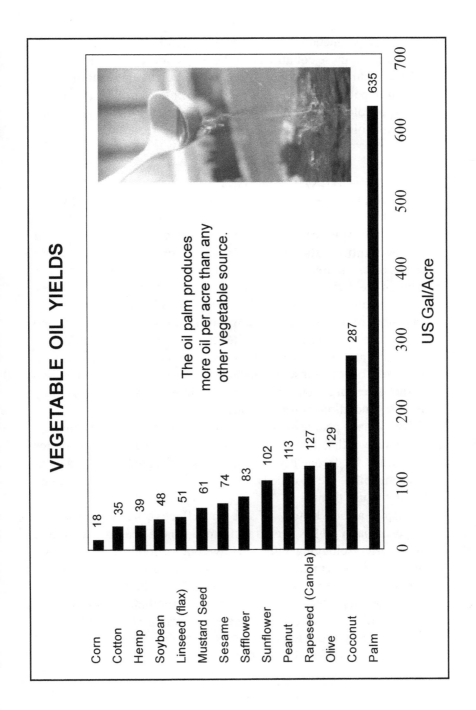

VEGETABLE OIL YIELDS

The oil palm produces more oil per acre than any other vegetable source.

Crop	US Gal/Acre
Corn	18
Cotton	35
Hemp	39
Soybean	48
Linseed (flax)	51
Mustard Seed	61
Sesame	74
Safflower	83
Sunflower	102
Peanut	113
Rapeseed (Canola)	127
Olive	129
Coconut	287
Palm	635

US Gal/Acre

Palm oil production is an important industry in Malaysia, Indonesia, and Nigeria. In these countries it is the major source of fat in the diet. The Malaysian diet has about 27 percent fat, eighty percent of which comes from palm oil. Palm oil is used all over the world. Virgin or red palm oil is sold as a health product and sells at a higher price than refined palm oil.

THE TROPICAL OILS SCARE

Palm oil has been a part of the human diet for thousands of years. Up until the late 1980s you could find palm oil in many prepared foods sold in North America and Europe. Manufacturers preferred it over other vegetable fats because it gave foods many desirable characteristics. In areas of the world where palm oil has been used as a staple in the diet, common illnesses such as heart disease, diabetes, and cancer have been relatively low, attesting to its healthful nature. It has a history of use as a healing salve for wounds and to ease pain and as a medicine to treat a number of health problems such as headaches, rheumatism, and cancer, and to improve reproductive health. Pregnant women went out of their way to include ample amounts of palm oil into their diet to ensure themselves a trouble-free delivery and a healthy baby. For generations it was considered a useful, healthy fat.

Today many people avoid palm oil, particularly in North America. Here the view is that it is an artery clogging saturated fat that promotes heart disease. We frequently hear warnings in the media to avoid palm and coconut oils—the so-called tropical oils. Diet and health gurus often tell us not to use them.

Despite a long history of safe and effective use, within a few short years, palm oil has been transformed from a healthy food into a despised artery clogging villain. How could a food that has served mankind well for so many years suddenly become a diabolical poison?

The answer to that question is a combination of greed, misunderstanding, and clever marketing. It has nothing do with science or with fact. The attack against palm oil was a cleverly designed publicity campaign sponsored by the vegetable oil industry in the United States as a means of increasing profits. Welcome to Marketing 101.

How do you convince customers to buy your product even though it is inferior to the competition? One way is to price it below the competition.

Another way is to lie. Years ago companies could get away with bold faced lies. Today there are laws that prohibit false advertising. Nowadays marketers use a new strategy—legal lying. Lie as much as possible without breaking the law. Even if your competitor's product is superior to yours in every way, if you can create the impression in the minds of the customer that his product is inferior, you win. How do you do that? Publicity! This is how the vegetable oil industry succeeded in taking over the tropical oils market and in so doing gave these oils an undeserved bad reputation.

The domestic vegetable oil industry in the US has been trying to capture the imported oils market for decades. At first their approach was based on price, but rather than lowering their price, they focused on getting the competition to increase theirs. In the 1930s they were successful in getting Congress to impose a sales tax on palm and coconut oils. Consequently, the price for these oils increased. Many customers switched to the cheaper domestic oils. This strategy worked for many years. Then in 1966 the tax was suspended and domestic oil producers had to compete on an even playing field. Several attempts have been made by the domestic vegetable oil industry to reinstate a tax on imported oils. To date these attempts have failed. A new plan of attack was needed—legal lying.

During the 1960s and 1970s heart disease was at an all time high. Elevated blood cholesterol was proposed as a possible cause. Saturated fats, in general, were being scrutinized because of their tendency to raise cholesterol.

Unlike other vegetable oils, palm and coconut oils were highly saturated. Vegetable oil industry executives reasoned that if they could instill fear and prejudice in people against saturated fats they could capture the tropical oils market. They mapped out a strategy to attack saturated fats and particularly tropical oils using heart disease as their battle cry.

Spearheaded by the American Soybean Association (ASA), the vegetable oil industry waged a vicious campaign demonizing saturated fats. Their aim was to create the image in the public mind that saturated fats are the cause of heart disease. Fueled by the ASA, the media began spewing out stories on the dangers of saturated fat and tropical oils. In 1986, the ASA sent out a "Fat Fighter Kit" to nearly a half million soybean growers encouraging them to write to government officials and food companies protesting the importation of the highly saturated tropical fats of palm and coconut oils.

Seeing the anti-saturated fat campaign as a means to increase their profits, the pharmaceutical and the weight loss industries joined in the attack. Special interest groups such as The Center for Science in the Public Interest (CSPI) and the National Heart Savers Association jumped on the bandwagon and started producing alarming news stories and advertisements attacking animal fats and tropical oils.

The CSPI, a staunchly anti-saturated fat organization, was especially aggressive in their attack on tropical oils. In 1988, CSPI published a booklet called *Saturated Fat Attack*. One section titled "Those Troublesome Tropical Oils," encouraged food processors to put warnings on their labels. CSPI apparently never took the time to actually study the issue and research the health effects of these oils. If they had done so, they would have found a wealth of information exonerating these oils from any wrongdoing. But in their zeal to condemn all saturated fats, they blindly attacked the tropical oils. Because of their limited understanding of fat and oil biochemistry, the booklet contained many errors and distorted the facts. Readers unaware of the shortcomings of the booklet were swayed against the tropical oils.

The media bombarded the public so frequently with anti-saturated fat, anti-tropical oil rhetoric that eventually everyone began to believe that palm and coconut oils caused heart disease. This anti-saturated fat campaign wasn't just an American battle; it spread throughout the world. Even in countries were the tropical oils were produced and widely used, people were frightened into believing the oils were dangerous.

Fueled by the relentless attack from the CSPI, commercial and consumer groups started lobbying the government to require a health warning on products containing tropical oils. Foods began to appear with the statement "contains no tropical oils" proudly displayed on the label. Tropical oil producers from the Philippines, Malaysia, and elsewhere, unable to match the financial promotional efforts of the soybean industry, protested the smear campaign used to attack their products.

In June of 1988 congressional hearings were held to settle the tropical oils issue. The domestic vegetable oil industry had their "experts" testify about the dangers of tropical oils. Lipid researchers not on the payrolls of the vegetable oil industry were also called to testify. Dr. George Blackburn, a Harvard Medical School researcher, testified that these oils do not have a harmful effect on blood cholesterol even in situations where they serve as the sole source of fat. It was pointed out that palm and coconut oils have been consumed as a substantial part of the diet of many groups of people for thousands of years with absolutely no evidence of any harmful effects. At the end of the hearings the evidence against the tropical oils didn't stack up, and no health warning went into effect. Companies who had begun using the "no tropical oils" claim on their products were told to remove the statement because it implied an unsubstantiated health claim.

Researchers familiar with palm and coconut oils couldn't understand all the criticism. Studies clearly showed that the tropical oils did not promote heart disease. If anything, they help protect against it. To all those who knew the facts about these oils, this was not a health issue at all, but a profit motivated publicity campaign. Dr. C. Everett Koop, the surgeon general of the US at the time, called the tropical oil scare "Foolishness!" and added, "but to get the word to commercial interests terrorizing the public about nothing is another matter."

The failure of CSPI and the vegetable oil industry to invoke a health claim against the tropical oils didn't stop them. They continued to condemn tropical oils as "artery clogging" saturated fats. People fell for it. Animal fat and tropical oil consumption declined and vegetable oil sales skyrocketed.

Restaurants and food producers sensitive to customer fear of saturated fats began removing tropical oils and other saturated fats from their products and replacing them with vegetable oils. Fast food chains proudly announced that they had switched to healthier vegetable oils for frying. By the early 1990s tropical oils had virtually disappeared from the American diet as well as the diets of most other Western countries. Even in countries that produced the tropical oils, palm and coconut oils were on the decline. Sales of soybean oil rapidly increased worldwide. CSPI proudly proclaimed its victory against tropical oils.

A FABRICATED HEALTH ISSUE

The entire anti-saturated fat campaign was designed to appear as a health issue. Polyunsaturated vegetable oils were promoted as healthy alternatives because they didn't raise blood cholesterol. When restaurants and food producers made the switch, the public assumed saturated fats were being replaced by "heart friendly" vegetable oils. What the vegetable oil promoters conveniently failed to mention was that the type of vegetable oil that was replacing saturated fats was anything but heart friendly. The oil that replaced the tropical oils was *hydrogenated* vegetable oil—the unhealthiest fat in the human diet. The public had been deceived.

Why were hydrogenated oils used instead of liquid vegetable oils? Liquid vegetable oils cannot replace saturated fats in food preparation and give the same results. Harder fats are needed to give foods the qualities customers expect. Hydrogenated vegetable oils are the only fats that can substitute for saturated fats. The vegetable oil industry knew this all along, but never revealed it to the public.

The problem with hydrogenated oils is that during the hydrogenation process, polyunsaturated fats are transformed into trans fatty acids— toxic artificial fats. By 1990 a number of studies were emerging showing that trans fatty acids promoted heart disease, diabetes, autoimmune disease, and a host of other health problems. "These are probably the most toxic fats ever known," says Walter Willett, M.D., professor of nutrition at Harvard School of Public Health. "It looks like trans fatty acids are two to three times as bad as saturated fats in terms of what they do to blood lipids."[1] Dr. Willett and his colleagues at Harvard University estimate that the consumption of trans fats in the American diet cause up to 228,000 heart attacks each year.

With the removal of tropical oils, hydrogenated vegetable oils penetrated every level of our food supply. By the early 1990s we were consuming*10 times* as much harmful trans fats as we had a decade earlier.

Consumption of trans fats ranges up to about 15 percent of calories, depending on a person's diet. Even tiny amounts of trans fats pose a threat. A mere 2 percent increase in energy from trans fatty acids increases risk for heart disease by 25 percent.[2] According to a report by the Danish Nutrition Council, trans fats are up to 10 times worse than saturated fats as a risk factor for heart disease. Dr. Willett says

18

that removing trans fats would probably have more affect than anything else we can do in preventing heart attack deaths.

The campaign to remove so-called unhealthy saturated fats and replace them with "heart friendly" vegetable oils was nothing but a scam. In their quest to gain greater profits, the soybean industry and their friends succeeded in removing harmless tropical oils from our diet and replaced them with a true artery clogging nightmare. You and I and everyone else are the victims of this deplorable scam. Hydrogenated or partially hydrogenated vegetable oils are found everywhere from baked goods and frozen dinners to baby food and dietary supplements. All of us are now exposed to this menace.

In 2003 the United States Institute of Medicine reported the results of a three-year investigation of all published studies on hydrogenated vegetable oils and trans fats. Their conclusion was that no level of trans fats are safe in the diet. This is interesting because the Institute of Medicine didn't give a limit that would be considered safe; they flatly stated that *no* amount was safe. According to them even the tiniest amount poses a health risk. As a result of these findings the FDA passed a law requiring the labeling of trans fats beginning in the year 2006. The FDA said this labeling requirement will encourage people to make better food choices which will prevent numerous deaths each year from heart disease. The FDA acknowledges that hydrogenated vegetable oils cause or at least contribute to heart disease, something that the vegetable oil industry couldn't prove with tropical oils, as revealed in the senate hearings a few years earlier.

TRANS FAT COVER-UP

After more than three decades of intense scrutiny by researchers attempting to prove that tropical oils are harmful, the oils have come out squeaky clean. Not only have they been proven not to promote heart disease, but evidence shows that they can protect against it.

Many of the studies done in the 1960s and 1970s which implicated saturated fat as a possible contributor to heart disease were actually done using hydrogenated vegetable oils, not saturated fats. Complete hydrogenation turns unsaturated fats into saturated fats. Most researchers thought that it didn't matter where the saturated fats came from so long as they were saturated. At the time they didn't know there was a difference between natural saturated fats and hydrogenated fats.

Hydrogenated palm and coconut oils were often used. People reading the studies ignored the term "hydrogenated" and simply associated palm and coconut oil with the negative results they were finding. It didn't matter if they used hydrogenated palm, coconut, or soybean oil, hydrogenated oil from *any* source raised blood cholesterol.

The detrimental effects of trans fatty acids were suspected as far back as the 1950s. Some researchers at the time even suggested that they may cause or contribute to heart disease. Research throughout the 1960s and 1970s also showed that hydrogenated fats produced a number of adverse health effects in lab animals. One of the primary concerns was the effect of trans fatty acids on essential fatty acid (EFA) utilization. Eating hydrogenated oils could cause EFA deficiency. One of the symptoms of EFA deficiency is elevated cholesterol—a risk factor for heart disease. Hydrogenated fats not only raise total cholesterol but also LDL, the so-called "bad" cholesterol, and lowers HDL, the "good" cholesterol. Trans fatty acids block prostaglandin synthesis which leads to hormonal imbalance, stunts testicular development in the young, and causes testicular degeneration in mature animals. Trans fats in the diet are incorporated into cells and alter composition of tissues throughout the body. Higher levels of fat accumulate in the heart, liver, and other organs. Trans fats retard kidney development, stunt growth, and interfere with blood sugar metabolism. Nursing mothers who eat hydrogenated oils pass trans fatty acids to their children through their breast milk.

Much of this was known and available in published studies by the mid 1980s, even before the vegetable oil industry started their anti-saturated fat campaign and their push to replace tropical oils with hydrogenated oil, explaining why industry representatives always alluded to replacing saturated fats with "vegetable" oil rather than "hydrogenated vegetable" oil. If the public knew that the vegetable oil industry was planning on using hydrogenated oils, they would have had a bigger fight on their hands.

The vegetable oil and pharmaceutical industries fund a great deal of research. Concerned about unfavorable findings that began surfacing in the 1950s and 1960s, they began countermeasures to show that hydrogenated fats were safe. They especially didn't want hydrogenated oils implicated as a possible cause of heart disease. They financed studies to show that hydrogenated oils were harmless to the heart and circulatory system. Negative findings were ignored and even suppressed.

Researchers depend on funding organizations to finance their work and advance their careers. Consequently, researchers try very hard to produce results that are favorable to those funding the studies. If they publicize results unfavorable to the funding institution, they may not receive support for future projects. So most researchers are highly motivated to produce good results and ignore unfavorable information.

Those who attempted to publicize negative effects are faced with the threat of no more financial assistance and complete ostracization from other funding organizations. When Mary Enig, PhD, a noted researcher and cofounder of the Weston A. Price Foundation, discovered the harmful effects of trans fatty acids, she ignored the normal protocol of suppressing the information and published anyway. Her financial sources withdrew their support and all future funding dried up. She was labeled a troublemaker and shunned by the vegetable oil industry. She was forced to make a shift in her career plans. The idea of a researcher searching for truth, regardless of the consequences, apparently no longer applies. The industry isn't looking for the truth; it only wants ammunition to use in their marketing. In other words, you play by their rules or you don't play at all.

The link between heart disease and trans fatty acids was suppressed for many years. Many researchers knew about it, but the general public was ignorant. Even though the vegetable oil industry was aware of the dangers of hydrogenated fats, they promoted shortening and margarine as healthier alternatives to saturated fats. It is very similar to the tobacco industry who denied that smoking caused lung cancer even when faced with overwhelming evidence to the contrary. Just like the tobacco industry, the vegetable oil industry suppressed studies and hid evidence. But as evidence linking lung cancer and tobacco mounted, so did the evidence against hydrogenated vegetable oils.

As studies continued throughout the 1990s and beyond, the true character of hydrogenated oil slowly emerged. Instead of being a heart friendly "vegetable" oil, it turns out it was more detrimental to heart health than any other fat. In addition to the conditions mentioned above, trans fatty acids are found to contribute to low birth weight babies, visual abnormalities in infants, childhood asthma, reproductive dysfunction, obesity, and lower immunity. If the consumption of trans fatty acids has caused you or your family to suffer from any of these conditions, you can thank the vegetable oil industry and their friends, such as CSPI.

THE BATTLE CONTINUES

The reason hydrogenated vegetable oils are added to foods is to improve texture and increase shelf life. Hydrogenated fats do not go rancid as quickly as liquid vegetable oils so they make suitable oils for frying in restaurants where oils are heated and reheated over and over again. Also hydrogenated oils can be heated to high temperatures with far less oxidation than liquid vegetable oils. Oxidation alters flavor and creates harmful free radicals. So what's the solution to hydrogenated fats?

The solution is simple. What did food processors and restaurants use before they had hydrogenated oils? Saturated fats. One of the best for cooking is palm oil. Now that hydrogenated vegetables oils have been exposed as health hazards, food processors are removing them and switching back to palm and coconut oils.

The transition isn't easy however. Many misguided individuals are fighting this change. The CSPI, backed by their friends in the seed oil industry, is actively campaigning against the used of tropical oils. Horrified that palm oil is now replacing hydrogenated fats in many commercial foods, the CSPI has renewed its attack on tropical oils, taking particular aim at the palm oil industry.

The CSPI is attacking individual food manufacturers for putting palm oil in their products, particularly those in the health food industry, calling them irresponsible for claiming that palm oil is a healthier choice. Palm oil, they say, is a saturated fat and saturated fats cause heart disease. This claim, however, has been soundly refuted by overwhelming evidence in published medical journals. Bringing this information to the awareness of CSPI should have convinced any honest truth seeker, but not the CSPI. They apparently are not after the truth but trying to win a campaign against saturated fats.

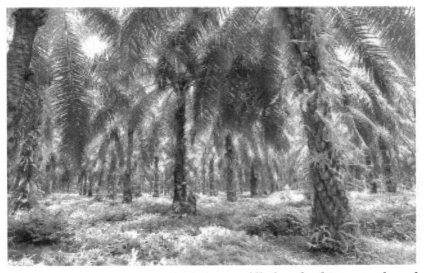

Palm plantations are like thick forests filled with plant growth and wildlife. After maturity trees remain productive for a quarter of a century. This allows the land to remain relatively undisturbed for years without disrupting the ecology. In contrast, soybeans and corn must be replanted each year with heavy applications of chemical fertilizers and pesticides.

Seeing that they could not attack the palm oil on the grounds that it promotes heart disease, they have resorted to other tactics. Reaching into their bag of tricks, they have began attacking the character of the palm oil producers. In an effort to sway public opinion against the palm oil industry, they began taking out full page ads in newspapers, such as the *New York Times*, claiming that these companies were destroying rainforests in Malaysia and Indonesia to make room for palm plantations. In clearing the jungles, the natural habitat of endangered species such as the orangutan, were in eminent danger.

The problem with this argument is that it is completely untrue. Again CSPI is deceiving the public. These countries have environmental and conservation laws in place now that protect endangered species and strictly limit clearing of jungle land. In Malaysia, for instance, the vast majority of the land used for palm cultivation over the last 20 years has come from preexisting rubber, cocoa, and coconut farms, or from logged-over forests in areas zoned for agriculture. Areas with endangered species are strictly off limits.

Over the past century forests have obviously been cleared to make way for cultivation and economic growth. This has been necessary to meet the demands from a growing population. *Every country in the world has done the same thing!* To focus on one or two countries and criticize them for doing this demonstrates extreme prejudice and lack of compassion. Many people in these countries are impoverished. Malnutrition and unemployment are high. To tell them they do not have the right to cultivate their own land so they can feed and cloth their people is absurd.

Malaysia is the world's primary palm oil producer, yet less than 19 percent of the country's total landmass is currently used for cultivation for various agricultural crops, including oil palm. This is small in comparison to the amount of land used in the United States and Europe.

Palm oil cultivation is more environmentally friendly than any other seed oil crop in the world. It uses only a fraction of the land area required by other oil crops, thus preserving forests and protecting the environment. Acre for acre, oil palm far out produces all other vegetable oil crops. For example, soybeans require 13 acres of land to produce the same amount of oil that palm can produce on just 1 acre. Corn requires 35 acres for the same amount (see table on page 13). In view of land usage then, which does more harm?

The land that is used for palm cultivation is utilized to the fullest with the least harmful effect on the environment. Wildlife is allowed to roam in and out of the farms unhindered. You don't see this on farms that grow soybeans, corn, or peanuts. Large animals would trample or eat the crops, so extensive fencing is required, further damaging the natural habitat. Soybeans require vast acreages of fenced off land. In addition, thousands of tons of pesticides are sprayed on soybean and other oil crops, causing untold damage to the environment, not to mention your health. Palm plantations generally do not use pesticides. So who is the more environmentally responsible? The answer is obvious.

Palm oil is not only produced under environmentally friendly conditions but it is also one of the healthiest oils you can eat. Replacing other oils in your diet with palm oil will help save the planet and your life.

Chapter 3

The Facts on Fats

FAT IS GOOD FOR YOU

Contrary to popular belief, fat is not some ugly beast that lurks in our food just to do us harm. It is a valuable, even an essential, nutrient. Simply put, fat is good for you. It nourishes the body and can help protect you from disease.

All natural fats are good. However, good fats can become bad if they are adulterated by man or consumed in excess. Some fats are better for us than others. Some can be consumed in larger amounts than others. Some need to be eaten in balance with others. Some fats, those that are adulterated or man-made, should not be eaten at all. The problem is that most of us are confused as to which are which.

Advertising and marketing propaganda has greatly influenced and distorted our perception of dietary fats. We are told to reduce our fat intake to the bare minimum in order to lose excess weight and be healthy. In addition, some fats are portrayed as being good while others are bad. Saturated fats, including palm oil, get the brunt of the criticism and are blamed for contributing to just about every health problem experienced by mankind. Polyunsaturated vegetable oils, margarine, and shortening, on the other hand, are hailed as the "good" fats. The truth is that most saturated fats, and particularly palm oil, are some of the healthiest you can eat. In contrast, many polyunsaturated fats are so far removed from their natural state and often chemically altered as to become a serious health threat.

Natural fats which have undergone as little processing and adulteration as possible are the most healthy, regardless of whether they are saturated or unsaturated. People from all walks of life and throughout history have been eating natural fats without experiencing the health problems we commonly face today. These fats are not the troublemakers.

Fats are, in fact, vital nutrients that our bodies rely on to achieve and maintain good health. We need fat in our diet. Almost all foods in nature contain fat to one extent or another. An adequate amount of fat is necessary for proper digestion and nutrient absorption.

Fats slow down the movement of food through the stomach and digestive system. This allows more time for foods to bathe in stomach acids and be in contact with digestive enzymes. As a consequence, more nutrients, especially minerals which are normally tightly bound to other compounds, are released from our foods and absorbed into the body.

Low-fat diets are actually detrimental because they prevent complete digestion of food and limit nutrient absorption. Low-fat diets can promote mineral deficiencies. Calcium, for example, needs fat for proper absorption. For this reason, low-fat diets encourage osteoporosis. It is interesting that we often avoid fat as much as possible and eat low fat foods, including non-fat and low-fat milk to get calcium, yet by eating reduced fat milks the calcium is not effectively absorbed. This may be one of the reasons why people can drink loads of milk and take calcium supplements yet still suffer from osteoporosis.

Fat is also required for the absorption of fat-soluble vitamins. These include vitamins A, D, E, K and important phytonutrients and antioxidants such as beta-carotene. Too little fat in the diet can lead to deficiencies in these nutrients.

Getting too much fat is less of a problem than getting too little. We are always encouraged to eat less fat because fat is believed to make us fat. This is just not so. Recent studies actually show that people eating the same amount of calories can lose more excess weight on moderate- and high-fat diets than they can on low-fat diets.

The amount of fat in the diet varies greatly around the world. Some people eat a lot while others relatively little. In many traditional diets such as that of the Eskimo, American Plains Indians, and the

Masai of Africa, fat historically comprised up to 80 percent of their total calorie intake (and the vast majority of it was saturated fat). Some Pacific island communities consumed up to 60 percent of their calories as fat, mostly from coconut, again primarily saturated fat.[1] Although these people ate large amounts of fat, it was natural unprocessed fat and modern diseases such as heart disease, diabetes, and cancer were completely absent among them. Relatively isolated populations that still eat natural fats do not experience heart disease and other degenerative diseases common in modern society.[2, 3]

In most countries around the world, fat consumption ranges from 20 to 40 percent of total calories. Health authorities often recommend limiting fat calories to no more than 30 percent. This limit is set primarily as a means to reduce risk of heart disease. However, studies on populations that consume over 30 percent of their calories from fat on average don't show any higher incidence of heart disease than those who eat less total fat.[4]

A healthy diet should include an adequate amount of good fat. The question that follows is: which fats are good and which aren't? The remainder of this chapter will give you the answers.

A QUICK COURSE IN FATS AND OILS

If you are already familiar with fatty acids, triglycerides, essential fatty acids, linoleic acid, alpha-linolenic acid and their function in the body, you can skip this section and go on to the next. If these terms are unfamiliar to you or you are unsure of their meaning, it will be of benefit to keep reading. This section contains a little bit of chemistry, but only a little. If you're not the scientific type, don't worry. My discussion here will be very basic and simple enough for the non-scientific person to understand. The main reason for this discussion is to familiarize you with some terminology that will help you understand fats and oils better.

The terms fat and oil are often used interchangeably. There is no real difference; however, fats are generally considered solid at room temperature while oils are liquid. Lard, for example, would be referred to as a fat, liquid corn oil would be called an oil.

Fats and oils are composed of fat molecules known as *fatty acids*. This is an important term to remember because we will be discussing

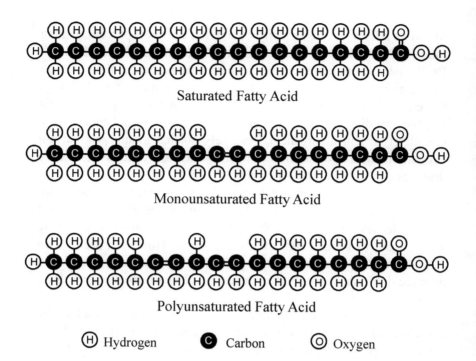

Saturated Fatty Acid

Monounsaturated Fatty Acid

Polyunsaturated Fatty Acid

Ⓗ Hydrogen   Ⓒ Carbon   Ⓞ Oxygen

fatty acids throughout this book. Fatty acids are classified into three categories depending on their degree of saturation. There are saturated, monounsaturated, and polyunsaturated fatty acids. You hear these terms used all the time, but what makes a fat unsaturated? And what are saturated fats saturated with?

Fatty acids consist almost entirely of two elements—carbon (C) and hydrogen (H). The carbon atoms are hooked together like links in a long chain. Attached to each carbon atom are two hydrogen atoms. A saturated fatty acid is one where each carbon atom is attached to two hydrogen atoms (see illustration). In other words, it is *saturated* with or holding as many hydrogen atoms as it possible can. Hydrogen atoms are always attached in pairs. If one pair of hydrogen atoms is missing, you would have a monounsaturated fatty acid. "Mono" indicating *one* pair of hydrogen atoms is missing and "unsaturated" indicating the fatty acid is now *not* fully saturated with hydrogen atoms. If two, three, or more pairs of hydrogen atoms are missing you have a polyunsaturated fatty acid. "Poly" indicating more than one.

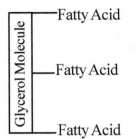

Triglycerides consist of three fatty acids joined together by a glycerol molecule. The fatty acids in our foods are in the form of triglycerides.

Doctors often use the term "lipid" in referring to fat. Lipid is a general term that includes several fat-like compounds in the body. By far the most abundant and the most important of the lipids are the triglycerides. When people speak of fats and oils they are referring to triglycerides. Two other lipids that are important in human health are phospholipids and sterols (which includes cholesterol).

The fatty acids in the oil you put on your salad for dinner and in the meat and vegetables you eat—in fact, the fat in your own body—come in the form of triglycerides. A triglyceride is nothing more than three fatty acids joined together by a glycerol molecule. So you can have saturated triglycerides, monounsaturated triglycerides, or polyunsaturated triglycerides. You can also have a triglyceride that has one of each fatty acid or any combination of the three.

All vegetable oils and animal fats contain of a mixture of saturated, monounsaturated, and polyunsaturated fatty acids. To say any particular oil is saturated or monounsaturated is a gross oversimplification. No oil is purely saturated or polyunsaturated. Olive oil is often called a "monounsaturated" oil because it is *predominately* monounsaturated, but like all vegetable oils, it also contains some polyunsaturated and some saturated fatty acids as well.

Generally, animal fats contain the highest amount of saturated fatty acids. Vegetable oils have the highest amount of polyunsaturated fatty acids. Palm and coconut oils are exceptions; although they are vegetable oils, they contain a high amount of saturated fat.

Some fatty acids are classified as being *essential.* What this means is that our bodies cannot make them so we must have them in our diet in order to achieve and maintain good health. Our bodies can manufacture saturated and monounsaturated fats from other foods. However, we do not have the ability to manufacture polyunsaturated fats. Therefore, it is *essential* that they be included in our diet.

When we talk about saturated, monounsaturated, or polyunsaturated fats, we are not referring to just three types of fatty acids, but three families of fatty acids. There are many different types of saturated fatty acids as well as many different mono- and polyunsaturated fatty acids. Two families of polyunsaturated fatty acids are important to human health; they are referred to as omega-6 and omega-3 polyunsaturated fatty acids. There are several omega-6 and omega-3 fatty acids. Two are considered essential because the body can use these to make all of the rest. They are *linoleic acid* and *alpha-linolenic acid*. These are the *essential fatty acids* (EFA) you hear so much about. Linoleic acid belongs to the omega-6 family. Alpha-linolenic acid belongs to the omega-3 family.

If you eat an adequate source of linoleic acid, the body can make all other omega-6 fatty acids it needs. Likewise, if you have an adequate source of alpha-linolenic acid, it can make all the other omega-3 fatty acids.

Getting enough linoleic acid (omega-6) is not a problem. Almost all plant and animal foods contain this fatty acid. Most of the fats we eat contain plenty of linoleic acid. It is the primary component of most vegetable oils. Soybean, corn, safflower, cottonseed, sunflower and other common cooking oils are predominately linoleic acid. Even canola oil which is referred to as a monounsaturated fat contains 22 percent linoleic acid.

Alpha-linolenic acid (omega-3) is less common. Flaxseed oil is a good source. A few other oils contain smaller amounts as do leafy green vegetables and seafood.

POLYUNSATURATED FATS
How Good Are They?

We hear a lot about how good unsaturated fats are for us. We eat soybean oil, safflower oil, and canola oil because we are told they are the "good" fats, the fats that will protect us from heart disease and other diseases. The problem is that much of it is a lie. It goes back to the marketing propaganda sponsored by the vegetable oil industry. We

COMPARISON OF DIETARY FATS

	Saturated Fats	Monounsaturated Fats	Polyunsaturated Fats
Safflower oil	9%	13%	78%
Sunflower oil	11%	20%	69%
Walnut	10%	24%	66%
Corn oil	13%	25%	62%
Soybean oil	15%	24%	61%
Cottonseed	27%	19%	54%
Sesame	15%	42%	43%
Peanut oil	18%	48%	34%
Canola oil	7%	62%	31%
Apricot	6%	63%	31%
Chicken fat	31%	47%	22%
Almond	9%	73%	18%
Avacado	12%	74%	14%
Lard	41%	47%	12%
Palm oil	50%	40%	10%
Olive oil	14%	77%	9%
Beef fat	52%	44%	4%
Butter	66%	30%	4%
Palm kernel oil	82%	15%	3%
Coconut oil	92%	6%	2%

■ Saturated Fats   ☐ Monounsaturated Fats   ☐ Polyunsaturated Fats

31

believe that polyunsaturated vegetable oils are healthy because that is what we've been told over and over again by advertisers and the media. Most people have bought into this lie. After all, if you hear a lie often enough, you will begin to believe it.

What consumers don't know is that polyunsaturated vegetable oils can be more harmful than saturated fats. Over the past two decades mountains of research have confirmed this fact. You don't hear much about this because companies can't make money reporting and publicizing negative findings on their products. That's just not good business. The vegetable oil and food industries are very good at promoting positive results of studies, yet they conveniently ignore anything that is negative. Consequently, the public gets a distorted view of the health aspects of polyunsaturated oils.

The American Heart Association and other health organizations have recommended that we limit our fat consumption to 30 percent of total calories consumed. Most people would assume that out of this 30 percent of fat calories as little as possible should come from saturated fat. Some say we need no saturated fat at all in our diet. That would mean the 30 percent of fat calories would need to come from monounsaturated and polyunsaturated oils. But did you know that researchers have found that the consumption of polyunsaturated oil exceeding only 10 percent of total calories can lead to blood disorders, cancer, liver damage, and vitamin deficiencies?[5]

Ten percent of total calories isn't much. If you replace the saturated fats in your diet with polyunsaturated fats, as is commonly recommended, you can easily get over 10 percent. And that could be dangerous! Let's look at what researchers are discovering about polyunsaturated fats.

Polyunsaturated vegetable oils lower our resistance to infectious disease by depressing the immune system. This fact is very well known. Vegetable oil emulsions are used for intravenous injection, for the specific purpose of suppressing immunity in transplant patients so that their bodies will not reject the new organ.[6] One of the ways polyunsaturated fats hinder the immune system is by killing white blood cells.[7] The white blood cells, which defend us against harmful microorganisms and cancerous cells, are the primary component of our immune system.

It is our immune system that is our primary defense against cancer. It has been known for years that polyunsaturated fats promote the growth of cancer.[8, 9] For instance, in one study conducted at the University of Western Ontario, ten different fats of varying degrees of saturation were studied to see how they affect the development of cancer. The animals in the study were fed the same diet differing only in the type of fat. Tumors were chemically induced in the animals. Those animals that developed the most and the largest tumors were those given polyunsaturated oils in their diet. The animals given saturated fats were remarkably resistant to tumor development.

The ability of high polyunsaturated fat diet enhancing chemically induced tumors has been widely reported.[10] Population studies also show that high polyunsaturated fat diets increase cancer risk.[11] Epidemiological studies demonstrate that dietary polyunsaturated fats can have a profound effect on cancer risk. Some researchers feel that cancer won't even occur unless polyunsaturated oils are included in the diet.[12] In other words, remove polyunsaturated fats and your risk of cancer plummets.

Heart disease has also been linked to polyunsaturated oils. This is of particular interest because most people associate saturated fat with heart disease, not vegetable oils. Studies have shown that both soybean and canola oils consisting of 20 percent of calories in the diet damages the heart causing heart lesions. However, adding saturated fat into the diet protects the heart from developing lesions.[13] It is interesting that you don't often hear about these types of studies. The vegetable oil industry isn't about to reveal the dangers of their own products. These types of studies are conveniently ignored and quickly forgotten. However, studies like these have prompted government agencies to recommend limiting polyunsaturated vegetable oil consumption to no more than 10 percent of total calories.

Polyunsaturated vegetable oils that we use every day such as soybean oil, corn oil, safflower oil—as well as margarine and shortening—promote heart disease. Linoleic acid, the primary fatty acid in these vegetable oils, increases inflammation, elevates blood pressure, and encourages blood clotting, all of which are risk factors for heart disease. In fact, the detrimental effects caused by linoleic acid are far worse than those attributed to saturated fat.

The incidence of asthma, eczema, and allergic rhinitis has greatly increased since the 1980s. This parallels the decline in saturated fat consumption and the increase use of polyunsaturated fats. Some researchers attribute the dramatic rise in these conditions directly to the increase use of polyunsaturated oils in our diet.[14]

The type of fatty acids in our diet determines the type of materials that go into building the cells in our brains and nervous system. Sixty percent of our brain is composed of fat and over half of that is saturated fat. Too much of the wrong type of fat in the diet can result in alterations in membrane fluidity, enzyme activity, and the binding of neurotransmitters and hormones to membrane receptors. When this happens, it can impair brain functions such as learning ability, memory, cognitive functions, and behavior. This may explain, at least in part, the increase over the past few decades in diseases that affect the brain such as Alzheimer's disease, Parkinson's disease, senile dementia, dyslexia, and perhaps even attention deficit disorder (ADD).

Several studies have shown the relationship between vegetable oil consumption and damage to the central nervous system. In one study, for example, the effect of dietary oils on the mental ability of rats was determined by analyzing the animal's maze-learning abilities. Different oils were added to the rats' food. The study was initiated after rats had aged considerably, allowing enough time for the effects of the oils to become measurable. Rats were tested on the number of maze errors they made. The animals that performed the best and retained their mental capacities the longest were the ones fed saturated fats. The ones given polyunsaturated oils lost their mental abilities the quickest.[15]

Age-related macular degeneration is the most common cause of blindness in the US, Canada, Australia, and most other industrialized countries. The incidence of this condition has skyrocketed over the past 30 years. Several studies have shown that the primary culprit in causing this rise in macular degeneration is the increased consumption of unsaturated vegetable oils.[16-18]

Polyunsaturated vegetable oil consumption has also been linked to the development of allergies, psoriasis, defective blood glucose regulation, migraine headaches, and a variety of autoimmune and inflammatory conditions including rheumatoid arthritis, irritable bowel syndrome, multiple sclerosis, lupus nephritis, and certain inflammatory kidney conditions.

So why hasn't the public been informed about the dangers of polyunsaturated fat? A few people have voiced concern about vegetable oils, but the food, drug, and supplement industries have been so successful in condemning saturated fat as the bad guy and promoting their products as healthy alternatives, we've all become brainwashed.

The fact of the matter is, researchers know about the dangers, but consumers don't. The reason is that most people get their health education from the advertising and marketing efforts of big business. Even the health food industry conveniently ignores unfavorable findings and emphasizes the favorable in such a way as to make a "questionable" product appear better. All businesses do this to some degree. The food industry is no different. Look at how the tobacco and drug industries have misled consumers for years about the health effects of their products in order to protect their sales. Do you remember the anti-inflammatory drug Vioxx? The makers of this drug hid information from the government and the public about the dangers of their product. Only after numerous heart attack deaths did an investigation reveal the truth. An independent study showed that those taking Vioxx had a five-fold increase in heart attacks and strokes. The drug was pulled off the market to avoid any additional deaths.

The food industry wants to sell products, so they will naturally publicize any positive research. Negative effects are doctored to make them sound less harmful or they are completely ignored all together.

Lipid Peroxidation

One of the reasons why polyunsaturated fats have the potential to cause so many health problems is because they are highly vulnerable to oxidation. When polyunsaturated fats oxidize, they become toxic. Oxidized fats are rancid fats. Free radicals are a product of oxidation. Free radicals are highly reactive molecules that destroy other molecules. When a free radical attacks another molecule it turns that molecule into a free radical, setting off a chain reaction that can affect thousands of molecules.

When oxygen reacts normally with a compound, the compound becomes "oxidized" and the process is called oxidation. However, under certain conditions, oxygen can react in such a way that an extra oxygen atom is involved in the reaction. When this occurs, the compound becomes peroxidized and the process is called "peroxidation." When polyunsaturated fats are oxidized, the process is called "lipid peroxidation." In this book I use the terms oxidation and lipid peroxidation in reference to the destructive oxidative reactions that cause polyunsaturated fatty acids to form free radicals and other toxic compounds.

Lipid peroxidation and the production of destructive free radicals is associated with cellular damage and dysfunction and is implicated as a cause or at least a contributing factor in many common health problems.[19, 20] Lipid peroxidation is a primary factor associated with heart disease, cancer, and the aging process.[21]

PubMed (an Internet database of medical studies used by researchers) lists over 32,000 published studies involving lipid peroxidation. So it is not an obscure process or theory. It is a well studied fact. And the fact is polyunsaturated fats when oxidized cause lipid peroxidation which promotes destructive processes in the body.

When polyunsaturated oils are exposed to heat, light, or oxygen, they spontaneously oxidize and form destructive free radicals. Once they are formed, free radicals can attack unsaturated fats and proteins, causing them to become oxidized and generate more free radicals. It is a self perpetuating process.

When oil is extracted from seeds, the oxidation process is set in motion. The more the oil is exposed to heat, light, and oxygen, the more oxidized it becomes. By the time the oil is processed and bottled, it has already become oxidized to some extent. As it sits in the warehouse, the back of a truck, in the grocery store, and in your kitchen cabinet, it is continuing to oxidize. In one study, various oils obtained off the shelf from local stores were tested for oxidation of the polyunsaturated fatty acids.[22] The researchers found that oxidation was already present in every sample tested. Those that had chemical preservatives added showed less oxidation than those preserved with vitamin E or other natural preservatives. When you use these oils in cooking, oxidation is greatly accelerated. This is why you should never cook foods using any polyunsaturated oil. This is also why when food processors removed saturated fats from their products they had to replace them with hydrogenated vegetable oils rather than ordinary vegetable oils.

Oxidation occurs inside our bodies as well. Our only defense against free radicals is antioxidants. Antioxidants stop the chain reaction which creates new free radicals. If we consume too much polyunsaturated fat, the free radicals they create deplete antioxidant nutrients such as vitamins A, C, and E as well as zinc and selenium and can actually *promote* nutrient deficiencies and all the numerous health problems associated with them.

Polyunsaturated fats are found in all of our cells to one degree or another. A polyunsaturated fatty acid in a cell membrane attacked by a free radical will oxidize and become a free radical and attack neighboring molecules, likely in the same cell. The destructive chain reaction continues until the cell is severely crippled or utterly destroyed. Random free-radical reactions throughout the body occurring day after day, year after year takes it toll. Is it any wonder why polyunsaturated fat consumption is linked to so many health problems?

In contrast, saturated fats are very resistant to oxidation. They do not form destructive free radicals. In fact, they can act as protective antioxidants because they prevent oxidation and the formation of free radicals. A diet high in protective saturated fats can help prevent lipid peroxidation that accelerates aging and promotes disease.

Polyunsaturated fatty acids are very easily oxidized. Saturated fatty acids are very resistant to oxidization. Monounsaturated fatty acids are in between. They are more stable that polyunsaturated fatty acids but less stable than saturated fatty acids.

Replacing polyunsaturated fats with saturated and monounsaturated fats in the diet can help reduce the risks associated with free radicals. Also, eating a diet rich in antioxidant nutrients such as vitamin E and beta-carotene will help protect the polyunsaturated fatty acids in your body from oxidation.

Heat Damaged Vegetable Oils

Most cooks recommend polyunsaturated vegetable oils in cooking and food preparation as a "healthy" alternative to butter, palm oil, or other saturated fats. Ironically, these unsaturated vegetable oils when used in cooking form a variety of toxic compounds that are far more damaging to health than any saturated fat could be. As it turns out, polyunsaturated vegetable oils are the least suitable for cooking.[23]

When vegetable oils are heated, these unstable polyunsaturated fatty acids are easily transformed into harmful compounds including a particularly insidious compound known as 4-hydroxy-trans-2-nonenal (HNE). When you cook with polyunsaturated oils, your food is littered with these toxic substances.

Even heating these oils at low temperatures causes damage to the delicate chemical structure of polyunsaturated fatty acids. Cooking foods at high temperatures accelerates oxidation and harmful chemical reactions. Numerous studies, in some cases published as early as the 1930s, have reported on the toxic effects of consuming heated vegetable oils.[24]

Over the past 20 years an increasing number of studies have found links between HNE and increased risks for heart disease, stroke, Parkinson's disease, Alzheimer's disease, Huntington's disease, liver problems, osteoarthritis, and cancer. Every time you use unsaturated vegetable oils for cooking or baking, you are creating HNE. Researcher A. Saari Csallany, a professor of food chemistry and nutritional biochemistry at the University of Minnesota calls it, "a very toxic compound." Based on her studies she recommends that people avoid *all* foods cooked in polyunsaturated vegetable oils.

One of the conditions linked to HNE in heated vegetable oils is heart disease. This may come as a surprise to most people because polyunsaturated vegetable oils are suppose to be heart friendly, yet recent studies show a clear link between HNE and heart disease.[25-27]

Studies show that diets containing heat-treated liquid vegetable oils produce more atherosclerosis (hardening of the arteries) than those containing unheated vegetable oil.[28] Any unsaturated vegetable oil can become toxic when heated. And even a small amount, especially if eaten frequently over time, will affect your health. Oxidized oils have been found to induce damage to interstitial tissues and blood vessel walls and cause numerous organ lesions in animals. Researchers are now beginning to recognize that heated vegetable oils are far more harmful to the heart and circulatory system than excess cholesterol or animal fats.

The oils that are most vulnerable to the damage caused by heating are the ones that contain the highest amount of polyunsaturated fatty acids. Monounsaturated fatty acids are chemically more stable and can withstand higher temperatures, yet they too can be oxidized and form toxic byproducts if heated to high temperatures. Saturated fatty acids are very heat stable and can withstand relatively high temperatures without oxidation. Therefore, saturated fats are the safest to use for day-to-day cooking and baking.

SATURATED FAT
The Saturated Fat Myth

Saturated fat has been blamed for more health problems than any other food ingredient on the planet. The words "saturated fat" conjure up visions of clogged arteries, obesity, and poor health. Doctors warn us not to eat it. Government agencies encourage us to avoid it. Everyone seems to criticize it, equating it to cyanide or arsenic—or so it seems.

But if saturated fat was as detrimental or as toxic as we are led to believe, why is it in just about everything we eat? Almost all foods in nature contain saturated fat. Meat, milk, and eggs contain the largest amount but saturated fats are also found in nuts, seeds, grains, and beans. Even broccoli, carrots, and peas contain some saturated fat. If saturated fat was so toxic, why has nature put it in just about everything we eat? Are the foods that nature has provided to nourish our bodies also designed to kill us? I don't think so.

The truth of the matter is that saturated fat is a vital nutrient. Yes, saturated fat is a *nutrient*, not a poison. It is necessary in order to obtain and maintain good health. Saturated fat serves as an important source of energy for the body and aids in the absorption of vitamins and minerals. As a food ingredient, fat provides taste, consistency, and stability and helps us feel full. Saturated fat is necessary for proper growth, repair, and maintenance of body tissues. Saturated fat is essential for good lung function. It is the preferred source of energy for the heart muscle. It also helps protect the unsaturated fats in your body against the destructive action of free radicals.

If you could see all the fat in your body, you would find that you are saturated with it. Every cell in your body contains fat. Saturated fat is an essential structural component of your cells. Your cell membranes consist of at least 50 percent saturated fat. Saturated fats are good and necessary for optimal health.

Probably no food component in history has been as misunderstood and maligned as saturated fat. It is labeled the cause of nearly every health problem of modern civilization. If it really is as dangerous as they say, it's truly a miracle how our ancestors survived for thousands of years eating a diet dominated by saturated fat. Animal fats, butter, and palm and coconut oils were the most common fats used throughout history. These fats are easy to produce using the simplest of tools. Vegetable oils from seeds such as soybeans, cottonseed, safflower seeds, and such are very difficult to extract. Consequently, polyunsaturated oils were not used much until after the invention of hydraulic oil presses near the end of the 19th century. Interestingly enough, when people ate primarily saturated fats, the so-called diseases of modern civilization—heart disease, cancer, diabetes, and the like were uncommon. Nowadays as we've replaced saturated fats with unsaturated oils these diseases have come upon us like a plague. From a historical point of view it is easy to see that saturated fats don't cause these diseases.

The primary reason why saturated fats are criticized is because some of them can raise cholesterol levels. Elevated cholesterol is believed to promote heart disease. In fact, thanks to the anti-saturated fat marketing efforts of the vegetable and pharmaceutical industries, most people believe that high cholesterol is the primary cause of heart disease. However, this is not true. High cholesterol does not cause heart disease. High cholesterol is only a marker or sign of increased risk of heart disease, not the cause. There are many risk factors. Being male or being physically inactive, for instance, are also risk factors but they don't cause heart disease. Our fear of saturated fat is mostly a man-made concept created to sell more vegetable oils and push cholesterol-lowering drugs.

Saturated Fat is Essential

We hear a lot about the importance of the essential fatty acids (EFA). Essential fatty acids are polyunsaturated fats. They are called "essential" because the body cannot make them from other nutrients so it is essential that we get them in our diet. Because they are called "essential" we get the mistaken belief that they are the most important fats. However, the reason they are "essential" is because they are the *least* important of the fats. Believe it or not, saturated fat is far more important to your health than the EFAs! Let me explain why.

Saturated fat is so important and so necessary to your health that our bodies have been programmed to make it out of other nutrients. Getting an adequate amount of saturated fat is so important to our health that it is not left to chance. The consequences of a saturated fat deficiency are so serious that the body is capable of manufacturing its own.

The EFAs, on the other hand, are far less important to our health, so the body has not developed a means of manufacturing its own. It relies totally on what is in the diet and has done so as far back as humans have existed. The need for essential fatty acids is so much less than that of saturated fat that the body can get all it needs totally from the diet.

Researchers tell us that we need about 3 percent of total calories as EFA. That is very small amount. As noted earlier, polyunsaturated fats (EFA) in excess of 10 percent of calories ignites a variety of health problems. Therefore, polyunsaturated fat intake of about 5 percent would easily prevent EFA deficiency yet not be so much that it causes problems. Dietary recommendations suggest a total fat intake of 30 percent of calories. If 5 percent comes from EFA (polyunsaturated fats) then where is the other 25 percent going to come from? Obviously it must come from a mixture of saturated and monounsaturated fats. This corresponds remarkable close to the fat profile of our bodies. The fat that makes up our bodies consists of 45 percent saturated fat, 50 percent monounsaturated fat, and only 5 percent polyunsaturated fat. That's right. Only 5 percent of the fat in your body is polyunsaturated. Our body's need for polyunsaturated fat or EFA is very small.

The fact of the matter is, your body needs a far greater amount of saturated and monounsaturated fat than polyunsaturated fat. You could live longer without EFA than you could without saturated fat. Your body needs nearly 10 times as much saturated fat as it does EFA. So which one is more essential?

Some people may argue that since saturated fat (as well as monounsaturated fat) can be made by the body from other fats and carbohydrates that we don't need to have them in our diet. Relying totally on the body to manufacture all the saturated fat we need would create a great deal of stress and cause a fatty acid imbalance. Researchers are learning that too little saturated fat in the diet can adversely affect health.[29, 30]

Palm oil makes an ideal all-purpose dietary oil. Its fatty acid content is remarkably similar to that of the human body—50 percent saturated, 40 percent monounsaturated, and 10 percent polyunsaturated. Thus it provides a natural balance of all three fat types. It's high saturated and monounsaturated fat and low polyunsaturated content makes it very heat stable and, therefore, an excellent cooking oil.

Chapter 4

Red Palm Oil

A FUNCTIONAL FOOD

If you asked almost anyone what they knew about palm oil, the response would probably be a blank stare or possibly the comment: "It's a saturated fat." The fact is, few people know anything about palm oil. Even most doctors and nutritionists are in the dark. This is surprising because palm oil is the most commonly used vegetable oil in the world. It is used primarily in Southeast Asia and West Africa where it is the main source of dietary fat for millions of people. Most people in North America, however, know very little about it and generally avoid it because they think of it as an unhealthy saturated fat.

The notion that palm oil is unhealthy is completely inaccurate. In truth, it is one of the healthiest oils you can eat. In terms of health benefits and cooking properties, it is far superior to corn, soybean, canola, safflower, peanut, and other vegetable oils. There are literally hundreds of studies published in medical journals describing the health benefits of palm oil. Yet if you asked your doctor about palm oil, you would probably be told to avoid it. If you asked why, the answer most likely would be: "Because it's a saturated fat." The fact of the matter is your doctor probably knows absolutely nothing about palm oil. If he did, he would recommend that you add it into your diet rather than cautioning you to avoid it.

The health benefits of palm oil are truly remarkable. It is what nutritionists' describe as a "functional food." Functional foods are those foods that have health promoting and/or disease fighting properties beyond their basic nutritional content, foods that can be used to improve health and fight off disease. Another term used to describe functional foods is *nutraceuticals*. *Nutra-* refers to nutrition or food. So nutraceutical means a food which can be used therapeutically. This is in contrast to pharmaceuticals which are chemical based medicines.

REFINED AND UNREFINED PALM OIL

There are two major types of palm oil—red palm oil and white palm oil. Red palm oil is essentially unrefined or virgin oil. Like virgin olive oil, virgin palm oil is extracted without solvents or added heat. The process basically involves squeezing the oil from the palm fruit and filtering out non-oil particles. White palm oil, on the other hand, has been refined, bleached, and deodorized, sometimes involving added heat and high pressures. It is also known as RBD oil, signifying it has been refined, bleached, and deodorized.

Palm fruit is a dark red color. When the oil is first extracted from the fruit, it has a distinctive bright reddish-orange color and is, therefore, called "red" palm oil. Red palm oil is rich in phytonutrients and has a characteristic flavor and aroma. When red palm oil is refined, some of the phytonutrients, including most all of the red pigmentation, are

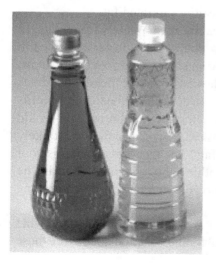

removed, leaving a light yellow, odorless, flavorless oil. Virgin or red palm oil, like virgin olive oil, is regarded as a premium quality oil because it is less processed and contains a higher nutrient content.

Palm oil has a fairly high melting point. At normal room temperatures the oil may be a thick liquid or a soft solid. On hot days it may be totally liquid. On cold days it may be completely solid.

Red and white palm oils.

In its solid state, refined palm oil is nearly pure white, thus the term "white" palm oil. When liquid, it takes on a light yellowish appearance. Red palm oil is dark red when liquid and a lighter orange-red when solid.

Both red and white palm oils have many uses and advantages over other vegetable oils. Red palm oil is of particular interest because it contains a rich source of health promoting phytonutrients that make it a powerhouse of nutrition. Some of these include carotenes (alpha-carotene, beta-carotene, gamma-carotene, lycopene), vitamin E (tocopherols and tocotrienols), vitamin K, sterols (sitosterol, stigmasterol, campesterol), phospholipids, glycolipids, squalene, phenolic acids, flavonoids, and CoQ10.

Red palm oil is one of the richest plant sources of cancer fighting squalene and heart protective CoQ10. It is the richest food source of two of the most important antioxidant nutrients—vitamin E and beta-carotene. Most notably it is the premiere source of tocotrienol, a highly potent form of vitamin E that is gaining recognition as a powerful anticancer, heart protective antioxidant.

Red palm oil is unique among dietary fats in that it contains the highest known concentrations of carotenes and vitamin E.[1] Antioxidants in foods prevent spoilage, as well as maintain flavor and nutritional value. These same antioxidants also provide significant health benefits. Antioxidants act to inhibit the damaging affects of lipid peroxidation reactions and free-radical production within the body.[2, 3, 4]

Palm oil has been used in hundreds of animal and human studies with no adverse effects. The safety of palm oil itself has been extensively evaluated and produces no physical or mental abnormalities and no evidence of toxicity even in extremely high doses. The old belief that it may be bad for the heart has been completely debunked. Palm oil, as it turns out, is not only heart friendly, but actively fights against the conditions that lead to heart disease.

Palm oil, and in particular red palm oil, is now gaining worldwide attention as a safe and important functional food that that can be useful in the fight against malnutrition, cancer, heart disease, diabetes, and many other health problems. In this chapter you will learn about some of the most important phytonutrients found in red palm oil and understand why and how the oil promotes good health.

VITAMIN E

Thelma Van Arsdel had taken vitamin E from the time she was in her early 50s until her death at age 93. The only time Van Arsdel stopped taking it was in her late 60s, and she said that during this time she began feeling the typical aches and pains of her age. But as soon as she began using vitamin E again, she regained her flexibility and was unusually alert and active the rest of her life. Like Van Arsdel, many people swear that vitamin E makes a dramatic difference in the quality of their lives.

Probably no other single nutrient has gained such widespread acclaim as vitamin E. In recent years, vitamin E has gained a reputation as a super nutrient and by some it has been hailed as a miracle vitamin. It is one of our most important aids in combating the effects of eating modern processed foods saturated with oxidized oils. Because vitamin E is a fat-soluble antioxidant, it battles free radicals within the fatty tissues of the body and is an effective warrior against one of our biggest health threats—lipid peroxidation.

A multitude of studies suggest that vitamin E provides some degree of protection from the effects of aging and degenerative disease. It has shown to be beneficial in protecting against cancer and heart disease as well as relieving symptoms associated with menopause; it enhances healing, prevents scarring on wounds, boosts efficiency of the immune system, improves sexual potency, and increases athletic performance, among other things. Benefits associated with vitamin E are continually being reported in the medical literature.

Vitamin E is an essential nutrient. A deficiency can lead to degeneration of red blood cells and anemia, muscle degeneration and weakness, and fibrocystic breast disease. Our white blood cells, the workforce of our immune system, require vitamin E to function in our defense against cancer and disease-causing microorganisms. Without adequate vitamin E, the entire body quickly deteriorates, accelerating the aging process.

A major factor in the efficiency of vitamin E in protecting us from the ravages of disease is its ability to act as an antioxidant. Vitamin E is found in every cell of our bodies. Here it functions as a bodyguard against renegade free radicals. Within the cell membrane (the outer covering or "skin" around our cells) it provides a first line of defense against free-radical attack. The cell membrane is composed predominantly of fatty acids, the *unsaturated* portion being easy prey to free radicals. When the body has enough vitamin E, this antioxidant is found liberally within the membranes of the cells. Vitamin E also patrols the inside of the cells protecting delicate organelles (cell organs) and DNA, both of which are highly vulnerable to oxidative destruction from free radicals.

A deficiency of vitamin E can leave cells without sufficient bodyguards to protect them, and the cells succumb to free-radical attack and quickly break down. It's no wonder why vitamin E has been labeled an anti-aging nutrient. Without enough of it, the cells and tissues in your body rapidly "age" as a result of the constant bombardment from free-radical invaders.

A deficiency can be caused by not eating enough foods with the vitamin, or excessive exposure to substances that generate free radicals. Vitamin E reserves are quickly used up in fighting free radicals and, if they are not replenished, our cells are left defenseless.

One of the most vulnerable places in the body to free-radical attack is the lungs. Air pollutants and some forms of oxygen, such as ozone, are strong oxidizing agents. Oxidation occurs when carcinogens react with polyunsaturated fats in our bodies, forming free radicals. Polyunsaturated fatty acids within the cell membranes of our lungs are readily exposed to oxidative elements in the air we breathe.

Free radicals play a key role in the development of all types of cancer. Lung cancer is the most deadly of all. More people die from it than any other form of cancer. One of the primary reasons why tobacco smoke is toxic is that it creates free radicals. Not everyone that smokes gets cancer, and cancer is not limited to just smokers. Nonsmokers also get lung cancer. Diet plays a big part in a person's susceptibly to lung cancer. Those smokers who do not get adequate amounts of vitamin E in their diet and consume lots of vegetable oil are the ones most vulnerable. Some smokers, knowing that vitamin E and other antioxidants afford a certain degree of protection against lung cancer, take heavy doses of antioxidant supplements; although it helps, a better option would be to quit smoking.

Vitamin E is a valuable aid in the fight against heart disease. Recent epidemiological surveys suggest that diets or supplements containing abundant vitamin E are of benefit in reducing the risk of coronary heart disease.

Since vitamin E is fat-soluble, its effects are most pronounced within the fatty tissues of the body, where you would expect to find cholesterol and polyunsaturated fat. Vitamin E protects these fats from becoming oxidized. Only *oxidized* fats are incorporated into arterial plaque. Normal fats are never associated with atherosclerotic arteries. If you have adequate vitamin E reserves, you are protected to some degree from the deposition of these fats in the arteries. Vitamin E helps protect arteries from free-radical injury that may initiate the atherosclerotic process and the development of plaque. Vitamin E also reduces platelet adhesion, thus reducing blood pressure and the tendency of blood to clot and clog arteries.

The World Health Organization conducted a study that compared death rates from coronary artery disease with several well accepted risk factors. The association between coronary artery disease death rates and elevated blood cholesterol was minimal. The best predictor of heart attack risk turned out to be low blood levels of vitamin E, and the lower the level the greater the risk.[5] According to this study vitamin E status has a much greater impact on heart health than cholesterol levels. You don't hear much about this because pharmaceutical companies aggressively market and advertise cholesterol-lowering drugs as the solution to heart disease and ignore inexpensive, natural solutions like vitamin E.

Vitamin E has been reported to reduce the incidence of heart disease in long-term users. In studies conducted by Richard Passwater, Ph.D., this vitamin's protective qualities were impressively demonstrated. The studies involved two groups. One group took 400 IU or more of vitamin E daily for at least ten years. The study involved 2,508 people from 50 to 98 years in age. Out of this number of people, statistical predictions indicate that 836 of them would develop heart disease. The actual number in this group developing the disease was only four, less than one percent of the expected number! The second group consisted of 1,038 people taking 1,200 IU or more of vitamin E daily for at least four years. In this group 323 would be expected to get heart disease. Only seven did.[6]

Numerous studies have shown that dietary intake of vitamin E either in foods or in supplements decreases risk of coronary disease by as much as 50 percent.[7, 8] Cholesterol-lowering drugs can't compare with this success rate. In fact, cholesterol-lowering drugs have only shown marginal benefit in preventing heart attacks.

Vitamin E has shown to have beneficial effects on certain diseases that are known to be associated with the over-consumption of vegetable oils. The autoimmune diseases lupus and rheumatoid arthritis are two examples. Studies also show promising results in slowing neurological problems in older people, preventing them in children, and in treating Parkinson's and Alzheimer's patients.[9] A study published in *The New England Journal of Medicine* put 341 Alzheimer's patients on daily regimen of either vitamin E or a placebo. For up to two years researchers charted the pace of the patients' deterioration. The result: those taking vitamin E showed a 25 percent less decline in mental ability. Research at the University of South Florida has shown that Alzheimer's disease is associated with free radicals. When these scientists added beta-amyloid, an abnormal protein that's one of the characteristics (and maybe a contributing factor) of Alzheimer's, to a lab slide containing blood vessels, it sparked the production of free radicals; these, in turn, constricted the vessels. In the brain, the same reaction would starve brain cells of oxygen and essential nutrients, killing brain tissue. When researchers treated the blood vessels with antioxidants like vitamin E, the vessels stayed wide open.[10]

Free-radical damage can affect brain function by limiting oxygen delivery to the brain, by contributing to atherosclerosis, or by damaging individual brain cells. In a series of experiments conducted by D. Harman and colleagues, mice were give different types of fat in their diet and their mental function was measured. When young mice were given oils containing vitamin E, they showed significant improvement in mental capacity over those fed oils lacking the vitamin. This demonstrated that free-radical damage, even at young ages, can affect mental capacity and that vitamin E can provide some protection against mental deterioration from free-radical damage.[11] It also demonstrated that unsaturated oils can promote free-radical reactions that affect brain function. Adding vitamin E prevents free-radical formation.

Vitamin E can give our immune system a boost to fight off foreign invaders and clean out dying and diseased cells. Jeffrey Blumberg, a human-nutrition researcher at Tufts University in Boston, tested the effects of vitamin E on the immune system of healthy older people. In a four-month study, different amounts of vitamin E were added to volunteers' diets. Each of 88 volunteers, age 65 and older, was assigned to one of four groups: members of the first group got 60 IUs (international units) of vitamin E per day; a second group got 200 IUs; a third got 800 IUs, and the fourth received placebos.

Although they theorized that vitamin E would produce positive results, what they discovered was startling. Normally, immune cells become less efficient as we age and don't protect our bodies as well against disease. But the cells of the vitamin E groups didn't act their age. "The responses of 65- and 70-year-olds looked more like those of 40-year-olds," Blumberg stated.

With results like those described here it's no wonder why people such as Thelma Van Arsdel, who took vitamin E regularly, lived to be 93. Like others, she found that the vitamin helped to prevent the typical aches and pains so often associated with aging.

The US RDA for vitamin E is 30 IU (10 mg). Many people don't get this amount. Commercial food processing destroys much of the vitamin E in our foods. People who consume a lot of processed and packaged foods can become vitamin E deficient. Eleanor Noss Whitney, Ph.D., R.D., former associate professor at Florida State University and president of Nutrition and Health Associates, states, "Processed and convenience foods do not contribute enough vitamin E to ensure an adequate intake." She further states, "A person's need for vitamin E is higher if the amount of polyunsaturated vegetable oils consumed is higher."[12] The reason for this is that polyunsaturated oils oxidize easily, especially when used in cooking. When these are oxidized, they form free radicals. Consequently, vitamin E is quickly used up or destroyed as it neutralizes these free radicals. Processed foods often contain oxidized polyunsaturated and hydrogenated vegetable oils, both of which can contribute to vitamin E depletion.

PALM TOCOTRIENOLS

Vitamin E is one of the major essential vitamins. Vitamin E, however, is not a single nutrient but a generic term referring to an entire family of eight closely related fat-soluble compounds. Vitamin E consists of two subgroups called *tocopherols* and *tocotrienols*. Each subgroup contains four members—alpha, beta, gamma, and delta.

Alpha-tocopherol is the form of vitamin E with which we are most familiar. This is the most common type found in our foods and the one in which the recommended dietary allowance (RDA) is based. Alpha-tocopherol is also the form of vitamin E used in most studies. When people talk about vitamin E they are generally referring to alpha-tocopherol. Until recently, it was considered the most important member of the vitamin E family because it was believed to be the most biologically active. Most dietary supplements use only alpha-tocopherol to the exclusion of all other forms of vitamin E. Recent research, however, has found that the often neglected beta-, gamma-, and delta-tocopherols also possess properties important to good health and work synergistically with alpha-tocopherol. Together they provide greater benefit than any one of them alone.

Tocopherols are by far the most common form of vitamin E in our foods. They are found in a wide variety of foods and most abundantly in vegetable oils, seeds, nuts, and grains. Tocotrienols, on the other hand, are far less common. In foods in which they occur, they are generally only found in small amounts. The sources with the largest amount of tocotrienols include wheat, barley, rice, and most abundantly, the fruit of the palm from which palm oil is extracted. Commercial quantities of tocotrienols are extracted from palm oil and to a lesser extent rice bran oil. Palm oil is by far the richest source of tocotrienols.

Eight Members of the Vitamin E Family	
Tocopherol	**Tocotrienol**
alpha-tocopherol	alpha-tocotrienol
beta-tocopherol	beta-tocotrienol
gamma-tocopherol	gamma-tocotrienol
delta-tocopherol	delta-tocotrienol

Palm oil contains both tocopherols and tocotrienols, making it a powerhouse source of vitamin E.

While tocopherols have gained most of the attention in the past, tocotrienols are emerging as the premiere form of vitamin E. Until recently, little research was conducted on tocotrienols because they are far less common. Initially, researchers didn't think they possessed much biological activity because after ingestion they only remain detectable in the bloodstream for 24 hours. It was believed that they were completely eliminated or metabolized within that time and, therefore, had little effect on health. We now know that they do not remain in the bloodstream for long because they accumulate in the tissues where they can have a significant impact on health.

As indicated earlier, tocopherols, especially alpha-tocopherol, are recognized as potent antioxidants and protective against numerous health problems. However, palm tocotrienols have proven to be more potent antioxidants and to possess superior overall health benefits.[13]

Tocotrienols are reported to have 40 to 60 times the antioxidant ability of alpha-tocopherol.[14] That means you can get the antioxidant benefit of 200 IU of alpha-tocopherol (the type used in most vitamin supplements) with less than 5 IU of tocotrienols.

One of the biggest challenges in the food industry is keeping food fresh for extended periods of time. This is of particular concern when food contains monounsaturated or polyunsaturated vegetable oils. These oils oxidize (i.e., go rancid) easily. Therefore, antioxidants are added to prevent oxidation and preserve freshness. Vitamin E (alpha-tocopherol) is a common food additive used to prevent oxidation of fats. Palm oil and palm tocotrienols are now being added to foods for this purpose. This is good news for us because it not only protects the food better, but provides us with this health promoting vitamin.

Tocotrienols are completely harmless. Toxicity studies show that tocotrienols are well tolerated and have no harmful effects even in large doses.[15] Unlike some other fat-soluble vitamins (i.e., A and D), no toxic effects are known with tocotrienol consumption, especially when taken in their natural form in red palm oil.

Researchers believe that tocotrienols, and even red palm oil, can have a significant therapeutic value for a number of health conditions. Palm tocotrienols can help keep our minds healthy by protecting the blood vessels going to the brain and maintaining proper circulation.[16]

Tocopherols and Tocotrienols

The terms tocopherols and tocotrienols are very similar and distinguishing between the two can be confusing. The vitamin E we are familiar seeing listed in dietary supplements and elsewhere are the tocopherols. In contrast, tocotrienols are the less common type found in palm oil.

The terms tocopherol and tocotrienol are used frequently in this book. If you don't remember which one is which, it can become confusing. A way you can quickly tell the two apart is the "tri" in the word "tocotrienol." Tri indicates the number three. Three of what? It is in reference to its chemical structure, but you don't need to worry about that, just think of *three* palm fruits. Whenever you encounter the word "tocotrienol" visualize the three palm fruits shown above. With this aid, you'll never get the words mixed up.

They can help protect against heart disease by preventing excess blood clotting,[17] protect against inflammation,[18] lower cholesterol,[19] and reduce atherosclerosis (hardening of the arteries).[20] Research shows they can protect against skin, breast, stomach, and other cancers.[21, 22, 23]

Vitamin E has been praised for accelerating the rate at which wounds heal. In animal studies wounds treated with vitamin E demonstrate faster healing.[24]

Aspirin is a common drug used to relieve pain and to thin blood. The primary drawback with aspirin is that it has a corrosive effect on the mucous membranes. With frequent use, as when prescribed by a physician to treat atherosclerosis, it can cause ulcers in the stomach wall. Since vitamin E has shown to be effective in speeding healing of cuts on the skin, it has been proposed as a remedy for aspirin induced lesions in the stomach. Studies indicate that both tocopherols and tocotrienols are effective in preventing aspirin-induced gastric lesions.[25]

Not only do the wounds heal faster, but scarring is reduced. Both tocopherols and tocotrienols possess anti-scarring properties. This characteristic has led to them being tested as anti-scarring agents in surgery, especially in glaucoma filtration surgery.[26-30] There is interest in using vitamin E in glaucoma surgery because it is less toxic than drugs presently in use. Mitomycin C, the drug that is most commonly used, is associated with potentially sight-threatening complications. In the search for a therapeutic alternative, alpha-tocotrienol and other forms of vitamin E have been investigated. Damaged cells (caused by injury or surgery) release substances that generate free radicals. Much of the pain and inflammation resulting from damaged tissue is a consequence of these free radicals. Vitamin E arrests the oxidation process, reducing inflammation and pain, and protecting against further oxidative damage. This also allows wounds to heal with less scarring.

Tocotrienols appear to be necessary for normal bone growth and calcification. In other words, without a source of tocotrienols in your diet, your bones can become weak. This is of major concern to many of us because as we get older our bones tend to lose calcium. Tocotrienols can help to keep them strong. Tocotrienols assist the body in calcium absorption, utilization, and deposition in bone. Tocotrienols are more effective than tocopherols in this process. In one study researchers compared the effects on bone building between tocopherol and palm tocotrienols. Supplementation with the palm tocotrienols improved bone calcium content, but supplementation with alpha-tocopherol alone did not. Investigators concluded that tocotrienols play an important role in the bone calcification process.[31] If you want strong bones, you should have a good source of tocotrienols in your diet.

Vitamin E supplementation appears to be effective in easing pain associated with arthritis. Vitamin E inhibits the elevation of free-radical concentrations associated with arthritis. It is the damage caused by free radicals that causes much of the pain. In a study on the effects of vitamin E on osteoarthritis, vitamin E supplementation was significantly more effective than was a placebo in relieving pain.[32] Another study of patients with osteoarthritis also showed that vitamin E was significantly superior to a placebo in regard to pain relief.[33]

Free radicals are believed to play a major role in development of cataracts, a leading cause of impaired vision and blindness in elderly people. Research has shown that vitamin E delays or minimizes development of induced cataract. The addition of vitamin E has a protective effect against cataract formation induced by radiation, glucose, or galactose. In rats made diabetic by the drug streptozotocin, there was extensive cataractous degeneration of the cortical cells within 6 weeks; vitamin E supplemented diabetic animals showed only slight lens changes. In an epidemiological study on cataract risk in adults over the age of 55, daily vitamin E or vitamin C supplementation or a combination of the two reduced cataract risk. Another study showed that subjects with high plasma concentrations of vitamin E have a reduced risk of senile cataract.[34]

Red palm oil contains about 600-1,000 mg/kg of mixed vitamin E. The vitamin E content is broken down into about 25 percent tocopherols and 75 percent tocotrienols.

VITAMIN A AND CAROTENOIDS
An Essential Vitamin

Vitamin A was the first vitamin to be identified by scientists in the early 20th century and, therefore, was given the designation of vitamin "A". It is an essential nutrient. We must have it in our diet to achieve and maintain good health.

Vitamin A is essential for good eyesight. One of the first symptoms of vitamin A deficiency is a decreased ability to see in dim light. This is caused by a decrease in photosensitive pigment in the retina of the eye, which requires the vitamin. A severe deficiency can lead to blindness. Not only is it required for the pigment in the retina, but it also helps maintain the health of the cornea—the transparent covering which allows light to enter the eye. Vitamin A acts as a protective antioxidant that helps to protect against lipid peroxidation which leads to cataracts and age related macular degeneration.

Vitamin A is essential for the normal growth and formation of bones and teeth in children. The vitamin is involved in laying down new bone during growth and in the formation of tooth enamel.

Vitamin A is essential for proper immune function. It is necessary to help fight off infections and protect against disease. A deficiency can weaken the immune system leading to frequent infections and increase vulnerability to cancer.

Vitamin A is essential for proper growth and tissue repair. After an injury, vitamin A is needed to help repair damaged tissues and protect against infection.

Vitamin A is essential for healthy skin and mucous membranes. The vitamin aids in the growth and maintenance of cells and tissues in the skin and the mucous membrane linings of the nose, eyes, digestive tract, lungs, and bladder.

Vitamin A is essential for normal reproductive function, oxygen transport in blood, and brain and nerve health. In short, vitamin A is essential for good health, and indeed, life itself. A deficiency of this important vitamin can have a pronounced impact on health.

Night blindness, caused by vitamin A deficiency, has plagued mankind for millennia. In Biblical times physicians treated the illness by feeding patients goat's liver—a rich source of vitamin A. Although they didn't understand why, they knew goat's liver cured the condition.

Vitamin A is a fat-soluble nutrient found naturally only in the fatty portions of animal products. The best sources are liver, whole milk, and egg yolks. It is not present in plant foods. Fruits, vegetables, nuts, and grains do not contain any vitamin A. When people speak of the vitamin A content in plant foods they are really referring to carotenoids, particularly beta-carotene. Certain carotenoids can be converted by the body into vitamin A. Beta-carotene, which is also referred to as provitamin A, has the highest conversion rate, approximately twice that of other carotenes. Most carotenes can't be converted into vitamin A at all. Conversion of beta-carotene to vitamin A is not very efficient. The US RDA for vitamin A is 5,000 IU.* You would have to eat three times this amount (15,000 IU) of beta-carotene to equal 5,000 IU of vitamin A.

Although plants do not contain vitamin A, they are the parent source of *all* vitamin A in our diet. Carotenoids in plants provide the basic building blocks for the vitamin A found in animal foods. The vitamin A you get in a glass of milk was originally beta-carotene in the grass that was eaten by the cow.

There are about 700 known carotenoids. Beta-carotene is the best known. Other important carotenoids include alpha-carotene, lutein, and lycopene. Carotenes are plant pigments that give fruits and vegetables much of their color. The red, yellow, and orange colors of tomatoes, carrots, sweet potatoes, squash, cantaloupe, mango, and papaya come

---

*Vitamin A amounts are indicated in international unites (IU) or retinol equivalent (RE); 5,000 IU equals 1,000 RE.

from carotenoids. Carotenoids, primarily beta-carotene and lycopene, give unrefined palm oil its distinctive dark reddish-orange color. Red palm oil is the richest natural dietary source of beta-carotene.

Carotenoids are not classified as vitamins because they are not considered essential nutrients. If they are not in your diet, you do not develop clearly identifiable deficiency symptoms like you would with a vitamin deficiency. That, however, doesn't mean they aren't important to good health. New research is continually being published demonstrating the importance of carotenoids in protecting against a number of degenerative diseases such as heart disease and cancer.

Beta-carotene is one of the most abundant and the most studied of the carotenoids. It is believed to be one of the most biologically active and the most important to human health. It is often added to foods as a coloring agent and as an antioxidant. Beta-carotene is vitally important for many populations around the world as it serves as their main dietary source for vitamin A. Many people cannot afford meat, milk, and eggs—the primary sources of vitamin A. Therefore, they must rely on beta-carotene from fruits and vegetables to meet their needs for this nutrient.

Beta-carotene and other carotenoids offer health benefits beyond their ability to be converted into vitamin A. Carotenes are potent antioxidants that can help protect against destructive free radicals. In this respect they are even more effective than vitamin A. Many of the carotenoids have also demonstrated anticancer properties with greater effectiveness than vitamin A. Beta-carotene improves the efficiency of the immune system by enhancing natural killer cell (a type of white blood cell) activity, which provides greater protection against infections, cancer, and environmental toxins.[35]

Although beta-carotene is the most well known and extensively studied of the carotenoids, it is certainly not the only one of importance. Other carotenes which include alpha-carotene, lutein, lycopene, zeaxanthin, and cryptoxanthin have therapeutic effects. Alpha-carotene has shown to drastically reduced the number of tumors in animal studies. The cancer-fighting ability of alpha-carotene exceeds that of beta-carotene. Lycopene, a pigment which gives tomatoes and virgin palm oil much of their red color, is being recommended in the treatment and prevention of prostate cancer. In one study, for instance, lycopene reduced the risk of prostate cancer by nearly 45 percent in men who consumed at least 10 servings a week of tomato-based foods. In contrast, those who ate four to seven servings a week had only a 20-percent reduction in their risk of prostate cancer. Lycopene has shown to protect against cancer of the mouth, pharynx, esophagus, stomach, colon and rectum. Lycopene is much more potent than beta-carotene in quenching singlet-oxygen, a type of free radical.

The greatest protection comes from a complete mix of carotenoids. Blood levels of total carotenoids were measured in 1,899 men and their cardiovascular health was followed for 13 years. The men with the highest blood levels of carotenoids had 36 percent fewer heart attacks and deaths than those with the lowest levels of carotenoids.

The dietary intake of several carotenoids in 332 lung cancer patients was compared to that of 865 cancer-free controls. After adjusting for smoking and other risk factors, researchers reported that the lowest risk of lung cancer occurred in those with the highest intake of mixed carotenoids.[36]

Carotenes can also help your body fight off infections by enhancing the efficiency of your immune system.[37]

Carotenes are often associated with carrots. Beta-carotene is what gives carrots their distinctive orange color. In fact, the name carotene was derived from carrots. Carrots are a good source of carotenes but they can't match the carotene content of red palm oil. Red palm oil has about 500-700 mg/kg of provitamin A carotenoids, which is 15 times more than carrots and 300 times more than tomatoes. Alpha-carotene (37%) and beta-carotene (47%) constitute about 84 percent of the carotenoid content in red palm oil with another dozen or so making up the remaining 16 percent.

Red Palm Oil Fights Vitamin A Deficiency

The idea that if a little is good, then a lot is even better is not necessarily true with vitamin A. Since vitamin A is helpful for so many potential health problems, it might be tempting to take large amounts. Mega doses of vitamin A, however, are not recommended. Vitamin A is a fat-soluble compound and, therefore, is easily stored in the fatty tissues of the body and particularly in the liver. If taken in excess, it can cause liver damage and other health problems. Getting too much vitamin

A from foods is rarely a problem, however. Synthetic vitamin A, the type used as a food additive and in most dietary supplements, is a much bigger concern. Synthetic vitamin A can become toxic at only moderate doses. Natural vitamin A, which is fat-soluble, is ten times safer than synthetic, water-soluble vitamin A.[38]

Some people have expressed concern about the possibility of getting too much vitamin A from eating carotene-rich foods. There is absolutely no risk of vitamin A toxicity from consuming beta-carotene. Beta-carotene is converted into vitamin A only in the amount needed by the body.[39, 40]

Because beta-carotene is safer to use than synthetic vitamin A, carotene-rich foods have the potential to help stem vitamin A deficiency. Vitamin A deficiencies are fairly common worldwide. In many areas, particularly in Africa and Asia, it is a serious problem. People who eat little meat or fat and rely on carotene-poor foods such as rice and other grains are the most vulnerable.

Vitamin A supplements can be used to prevent this problem. Supplementing the diet with a vitamin pill, however, isn't a prefect solution. Since the diets of populations in the affected areas lack adequate vitamin A, people would have to take dietary supplements for the rest of their lives. For many this is an expense they may not be able to afford. Some won't bother to travel to the medical centers on a regular basis to get the supplements. The danger of vitamin A toxicity is also a possibility. For instance, medical officials in eastern India launched a campaign in 2001 to provide children with vitamin A supplements. Many of the children were so deficient in this vitamin that workers gave them megadoses as high as 500,000 IU. Consequently, many of the children developed vitamin A toxicity and at least 30 died.

Giving people foods rich in beta-carotene appears to be a safer approach. Palm oil, being the richest dietary source of beta-carotene, offeres a possible solution. To test the effectiveness of red palm oil, studies were carried out to see how it compared with other sources of vitamin A.

In one study, researchers gave red palm oil or peanut oil fortified with vitamin A to preschool children in India. The study, which ran for a period of 7 months, was modeled to monitor the difference in the

Provitamin A Carotene Content (retinol equivalent)	
Food	**Relative quality (no. of times)**
Red Palm Oil	1
Carrots	15
Leafy Vegetables	44
Apricots	120
Tomatoes	300
Bananas	1,000
Orange Juice	3,750

Source: *Nutrition Briefs*, July 2004, Malaysian Palm Oil Promotion Council.

efficacy of the mode of supplementation and optimum dose of improving vitamin A status. Results showed that those children receiving red palm oil recorded more gain in vitamin A levels compared to the peanut oil/ vitamin A group. It was also found that as little a dose as 5 ml (1 teaspoon) was just as effective as 10 ml (2 teaspoon) given daily.[41]

The governments of Indonesia, Burkina Faso, China, Honduras, India, Nigeria, Peru, South Africa, and Tanzania have all successfully used palm oil to combat vitamin A deficiency.

Palm oil is a superior source of provitamin A then other foods, such as carrots and sweet potatoes, not just because of its high beta-carotene content but because it is a fat. Even if other carotene-rich foods were available, the problem might not be solved. The diet *must* also have an adequate amount of fat in order for the carotenes to be converted into vitamin A.[42] Carotenes are only converted efficiently into vitamin A when combined with fat. Low-fat diets either from choice or economic restraint greatly reduces the conversion of carotenes to vitamin A. Even diets with ample amounts of carotene-rich food will not prevent vitamin A deficiency if fat consumption is low. In Tanzania, for example, where a variety of carotene-rich fruits and vegetables are readily available and consumed, vitamin A deficiency is still prevalent because fat consumption is low.[43]

In countries where animal products are out of reach for economically disadvantaged people, the solution to the problem is to provide a source for both provitamin A carotenes as well as fat. Red palm oil lends itself exceptionally well for this purpose. The oil also improves the bioavailability of carotenes from other foods, making it an ideal solution to this worldwide problem. Studies in countries all over the world have proven that adding red palm oil into the diet is very effective in preventing vitamin A deficiencies.[44, 45]

Since vitamin A deficiency lowers immunity, disease and sickness can be significantly reduced simply by adding red palm oil into the diet. This was illustrated in a study in Indonesia involving 26,000 school children. Supplementing the diets of the children with vitamin A resulted in a 34 percent reduction in childhood deaths from disease. Therefore, adding just a little red palm oil into the diet can have a dramatic effect on the health of growing children.

In another study conducted in India, red palm oil was used in biscuits and given as snacks to children ages 13-15 years who had a history of repeated acute respiratory infections (ARI). One hundred children were given four biscuits made with red palm oil daily over 3 months. Fifty other children with a similar ARI history served as controls. The results showed that the prevalence of ARI decreased significantly from 38 percent to 17 percent. In the control group the ARI prevalence increased by 2 percent.[46] This study demonstrated that the use of red palm oil enhances immunity and helps protect against infections.

Palm oil also improves overall nutrient status and growth rate. In the above study those in the palm oil group, but not the control group had a significantly improved body mass index (BMI).

Vitamin A deficiency in pregnant and nursing mothers is also a serious problem which can lead to birth defects and growth and developmental problems. Adding red palm oil to a nursing mother's diet enriches breast milk with vitamin A and other nutrients important to the growth of the child.[47, 48]

Vitamin A deficiency is not restricted to just developing areas of the world; many people in more affluent countries are also affected. Junk foods, fast foods, and packaged convenience foods are all vitamin A deficient. Breads, rice, oats, potatoes, and many fruits and vegetables as well as vegetable oils contain little or no vitamin A or beta-carotene. The best source of beta-carotene comes from dark green, yellow, and orange fruits and vegetables, which most people don't eat enough of.

Even if you do eat plenty of carotene-rich produce, if you eat a low-fat diet you probably won't be getting the vitamin A you need because fat is needed to effectively absorb vitamin A. Eating a low-fat diet can contribute to the problem.

Consequently, many people do not get the minimum recommended 5,000 IU of vitamin A per day. In the United States vitamin A consumption averages only about 4,000 IU. Sickness, pollution, and stress increase our need for the vitamin. A marginal or subclinical deficiency produces symptoms that are mild and often ignored or misdiagnosed as simply part of the normal consequence of aging. Even a subclinical deficiency can cause serious health problems. Immunity is seriously affected by even a mild vitamin A deficiency, resulting in susceptibility to infectious diseases at two and three times the rate as those with normal vitamin A status. Adding red palm oil into your diet is a simple way of getting the vitamin A you need.

PALM SQUALENE

Squalene is a naturally occurring lipid which is structurally similar to beta-carotene. It is found in both plants and animals. The highest natural source comes from shark liver oil, with appreciable amounts in palm oil as well as olive, wheat germ, and rice bran oils. First discovered in 1906 by a Japanese researcher working with shark liver oil, "squalene" derives its name from the Latin word for the dogfish shark (*Squalus spp.*).

Studies suggest that squalene may be useful in treating cancer, strengthening the immune system, regulating cholesterol, and protecting against radiation and toxins. It is reported to improve appearance of the skin and hair, boost energy levels, improve circulation, and provide relief from arthritic pain, gout, and gastritis, among other things. For these reasons, it is sold as a dietary supplement. Whether it can do all these things is yet to be scientifically proven. However, studies do show that it may have some important health benefits.

Squalene is transported in the blood like other lipids and distributed throughout the body with the greatest concentration in the skin where it is one of the major components of sebum—the oil on your skin. Our bodies can transform squalene into sterols which can then be used to make vitamin D and hormones such as estrogen, progesterone, and testosterone. One of the sterols the body can manufacture from squalene is cholesterol. Oddly, even though squalene can be converted into cholesterol, it is being investigated as a means to *reduce* blood cholesterol. Consumption of squalene does not raise blood cholesterol levels even when taken in fairly large amounts.[49] The reason for this is that squalene consumption increases HDL, the "good" cholesterol, thus increasing excretion of LDL or "bad" cholesterol in bile acids, resulting in equalizing effect on total cholesterol and an improvement in the cholesterol ratio, thus reducing risk of heart disease.

Researchers believe squalene may be useful in the treatment of hypercholesterolemia (high blood cholesterol). Adding squalene to protocols using cholesterol-lowering statin drugs has been shown to enhance the efficacy of the treatment. For instance, the cholesterol-lowering effect of the drug pravastatin was compared to squalene. Subjects were divided into three groups. The first group received pravastatin (10 mg), the second squalene (860 mg) and the third a combination of both. Pravastation proved to be more effective than squalene alone in reducing cholesterol levels. However, the combination of both pravastatin and squalene reduced total and LDL cholesterol and increased HDL cholesterol better than each alone.[50] Doctors looking for more natural means to improve cholesterol levels can incorporate a good source of squalene, such as palm oil, into the diet of their patients.

Squalene is very resistant to peroxidation and, therefore, can be helpful in preventing the oxidation of less stable fats in the body. Acting as an antioxidant, it is very effective in stopping the action of free radicals.[51] It is comparable in strength to the synthetic antioxidant BHT, which is often used as a food additive.

When consumed, a large percentage of squalene finds it way to the skin where it makes up a significant proportion of our body's natural oil (sebum). About 12 percent of sebum consists of squalene. Squalene helps to moisturize and protect the skin and regulate surface environment. It plays a vital role in protecting our skin from the oxidizing and damaging effects of oxygen, ultraviolet (UV) light, and environmental pollutants. It has also been shown to help speed the healing of wounds.

Squalene is often added to skin care products because it is a good moisturizer and protects against UV radiation from the sun. It blocks the ionizing radiation that can damage the skin and cause cancer. In essence, it is the body's natural sun block and protective skin lotion.

As an antioxidant squalene is particularly effective in quenching the free radicals generated by radiation. Not just UV radiation but x-rays and other forms of radiation as well. Since squalene is dispersed to all tissues, it can protect the entire body from radiation, not just the skin. This was dramatically illustrated in a study in which mice given a diet supplemented with squalene were protected from lethal doses of radiation.[52] Mice not given squalene were exposed to whole body gamma-irradiation. They all died. A second group that were fed squalene were exposed to the same amount of radiation and all survived. By adding squalene into the animal's diet it increased survival rate from 0 to 100 percent. Those are pretty dramatic results!

What this means to us is that squalene may provide us with some degree of protection from various forms of radiation, not only just from UV light from the sun but from other sources as well. For example, consuming a source of squalene prior to getting x-rays or mammograms appears to be a smart way to help protect yourself from the detrimental effects of x-rays.

Animal studies have shown that squalene also plays an important role in the health of the eyes. Squalene is needed in the formation of photoreceptor cells in the retina.[53] The presence of squalene in eye tissue suggests a possible protective role against oxidative related vision disorders such as macular degeneration.

Another remarkable characteristic of squalene is its ability to act as a natural detoxifier, protecting the body from the detrimental effects of chemicals and toxins. Several intriguing studies have demonstrated the effect of the oral administration of squalene in neutralizing and eliminating a variety of toxic substances.[54-57]

Researchers feel that squalene is a good candidate as an antidote to reduce the toxicity of accidentally ingested drugs and poisons. In one study, researchers administered high doses of various drugs including theophylline, phenobarbital (a potent narcotic), and strychnine (rat poison) to lab animals. The animals were then fed squalene as an antidote. Squalene accelerated the fecal excretion and reduced blood levels of the poisons, thus providing the animals a significant degree of protection from the detrimental effects of these chemicals.

Squalene also blocks the cancer-causing effects of certain industrial chemicals and environmental toxins. A number of studies have demonstrated the anticancer effects of squalene in animals.[58-60] In one study, for example, lung cancer was chemically induced in lab animals. In the control group, which did not receive squalene, 100 percent of the animals developed tumors. In contrast, those that were fed squalene had 58 percent fewer tumors.[61]

Results of animal studies indicate squalene can suppress the growth of tumor cells, partially prevent the development of chemically-induced cancer, and cause regression of some already existing tumors. It also enhances immune function thus aiding the body in preventing and fighting cancer.

Several researchers have suggested that the observed reduction of cancer in human populations who consume olive and palm oils may in part be due to the relatively high concentration of squalene in these oils. Studies also show that squalene significantly improves the cancer fighting effect of chemotherapeutic drugs. For these reasons, the primary research interest in squalene is currently in cancer therapy.

There are no reported harmful side effects to squalene even in the relatively large amounts found in dietary supplements. One of the best natural sources of squalene is red palm oil. There are about 200-500 mg/kg of squalene in red palm oil. Using red palm oil as a normal part of your diet can supply you with a significant amount of squalene that can help normalize cholesterol, balance hormones, protect against oxidation, keep your skin healthy, preserve your eyesight, detoxify your body, block the damaging effects of radiation, prevent cancer, and strengthen your immune system.

PALM OIL COENZYME Q10
Essential for Good Health

Coenzyme Q10 (CoQ10), also known as ubiquinone, is a fat-soluble, vitamin-like substance present in every cell of the human body. Although not classified as a vitamin, it has been shown to be essential to health. A deficiency of this substance leads to nutrient related health problems. There are ten types of CoQ. CoQ10 is the most important in the human body. It is involved in the process of producing energy in the cells and, therefore, is vital to health. It also acts as a protective antioxidant. CoQ10 is closely related to vitamin E and works synergistically with it.

Although our bodies can synthesize CoQ10, normal levels are maintained by a combination of dietary intake and biosynthesis. A lack of adequate CoQ10 in the diet can lead to a deficiency.

CoQ10 is present in small amounts in a variety of foods. It is particularly high in organ meats such as heart, liver, and kidneys as well as sardines, mackerel, and the fruit of the oil palm from which we get red palm oil. Minor amounts are found in most meats because CoQ10 is synthesized in animal and human tissues as a necessary part of energy production. Red palm oil is probably the highest vegetable source for this important nutrient. For this reason, people who don't eat much meat can benefit greatly from adding red palm oil to their diets.

Although CoQ10 has been identified as an essential nutrient for optimal health, it is not classified as a vitamin because it can be produced in the body. The biosynthesis of CoQ10, however, is not an easy one. The complex process takes 17 steps requiring at least seven vitamins (riboflavin, niacinamide, vitamin B6, folic acid, vitamin B12, vitamin C, and pantothenic acid) and several trace minerals.

CoQ10 deficiency may be caused by a lack of this nutrient in the diet, impairment of CoQ10 biosynthesis in the body, excessive utilization of CoQ10, or any combination of the three. Decreased dietary intake can occur in malnutrition and chronic submalnutrition.[62] The nutritionally poor diets that are typical in the modern western diet can lead to CoQ10 deficiency and impair CoQ10 biosynthesis. Many people probably have suboptimal levels of this nutrient without knowing it.

Heart Function

CoQ10 is known to be highly concentrated in the heart muscle. This makes sense because the heart, one of the body's most energetic organs, beats approximately 100,000 times a day, 36 million times a year, and depends on CoQ10 for its energy needs. A deficiency of CoQ10, therefore, can lead to heart failure.[63] For this reason, most of the research to date on CoQ10 has been focused on heart disease. Heart failure from various causes has been correlated with low levels of CoQ10.[64] Severity of heart failure correlates with the severity of CoQ10 deficiency.[65]

CoQ10 has been shown to help heart function by enhancing the pumping action and electrical signaling, as well as helping to lower blood pressure. Clinical trials have shown that when CoQ10 is given orally to heart disease patients, heart function demonstrates gradual and sustained increase in volume of blood pumped and improvement in the patients' symptoms. The degree of improvement has on occasion been dramatic with some patients' hearts returning to normal size and function on CoQ10 alone. Studies have been remarkably consistent with no adverse side effects.[66-71]

In most studies CoQ10 was used in conjunction with standard medical treatments. Patients already had a history of heart disease and were taking medications as a part of ongoing treatment. The research has shown that with the addition of CoQ10, medications could be reduced or eliminated altogether. "The clinical experience with CoQ10 in heart failure is nothing short of dramatic," says Peter H. Lansjoen, M.D., a cardiologist and one of the leading CoQ10 researchers. "It is reasonable to believe that the entire field of medicine should be re-evaluated in light of this growing knowledge. We have only scratched the surface of the biomedical and clinical applications of CoQ10 and the associated fields of bioenergetics and free radical chemistry."

One of the risk factors associated with heart disease is high blood pressure. Elevated blood pressure can cause damage to artery walls initiating the process of plaque formation. CoQ10 can be useful in lowering high blood pressure. In one study, for instance, 109 patients on blood pressure lowering drugs were given CoQ10. Blood pressure gradually decreased in most of the patients, 51 percent of whom came completely off of between one to three blood pressure drugs after an average of 4 months.[72]

CoQ10 also appears to have a protective effect on the heart during chemotherapy.[73] Chemotherapy drugs, which are administered to kill cancer cells, often have a detrimental effect on many healthy tissues as well. The toxic effects on the heart are thought to be due primarily to free radical damage. Radiation therapy also generates a great deal of free radicals. CoQ10 being a potent antioxidant provides the heart with protection during chemotherapy and radiation therapy.

The antioxidant properties of CoQ10 reduce oxidative damage to artery walls and inhibit the oxidation of LDL cholesterol, thus reducing the formation of arterial plaque. So, not only does CoQ10 help protect the heart muscle itself, but it also helps keep the arteries open and healthy.

CoQ10 has been shown to be essential to proper heart function. All forms of heart disease can be adversely affected by a CoQ10 deficiency. Ironically, the statin drugs used to lower blood cholesterol in heart disease patients block the biosynthesis of CoQ10.[74] Cholesterol-lowering statin drugs interfere with the body's production of CoQ10.[75] Statins (i.e., prevastatin, simvastatin, lovastatin, etc.) inhibit a key enzyme involved in the body's production of cholesterol. However, the same enzyme is also necessary for the production of CoQ10. So when statin drugs block the body's production of cholesterol, they also stop production of CoQ10.

All of the cholesterol-lowering statin drugs that are currently being prescribed block the body's formation of CoQ10 and, therefore, *weaken* the heart. Blood cholesterol may be lower, but the heart is compromised at the same time. The heart uses a huge amount of CoQ10. "It has been pretty well documented from biopsies that the severity of heart failure correlates with the people who have the lowest levels of Q10," says Dr. Langsjoen. "I think people taking statins should be very worried. I don't think this can be ignored." Dr. Langsjoen has pointed out that people who live to 90 or more tend to have high CoQ10 levels. A good dietary source of CoQ10 can help solve this problem. Adding red palm oil, and other sources of CoQ10, to the diet would be a smart decision for anyone taking cholesterol-lowering drugs or for anyone concerned about the health of their heart.

Other Conditions

In addition to the heart muscle, CoQ10 is essential for the optimal function of all types of cells in the body. It is not surprising, therefore, to find a number of diseases which respond favorably to CoQ10 supplementation. Significantly decreased levels of CoQ10 have been noted in a variety of diseases in both animals and human studies, ranging from cancer and HIV to periodontal disease.

Abnormally low blood levels of CoQ10 have been reported in cancer patients.[76] This correlation is so strong that some researchers have proposed using blood CoQ10 levels as a means to evaluate cancer risk. Cancer patients given supplemental CoQ10 have shown remarkable improvement, with those receiving the largest dosages demonstrating the greatest effect. Several case studies reported in medical journals have documented complete regression of tumors in the breast, liver, and pleural cavity.[77, 78]

One of the ways CoQ10 helps to fight cancer is by enhancing the efficiency of the immune system. The health of the immune system is essential in combating infectious disease. As in the case of AIDS where the immune system is severely compromised ordinarily minor infections can become life threatening. HIV infected individuals have low levels of CoQ10. As levels drop, the severity of their condition increases. End stage AIDS patients have a significant CoQ10 deficiency. HIV attacks the white blood cells and destroys the immune system. Consequently, HIV/AIDS patients have an abnormally low white blood cell count. When CoQ10 is given to HIV/AIDS patients, their white blood cell levels increase.[79] This indicates an improvement in their condition and a strengthening of their immune system.

Another interesting aspect of CoQ10 is in the treatment of periodontal or gum disease. Periodontal disease is characterized by inflammation, swelling and oversensitivity and bleeding of the gums. Like other health issues, periodontal disease is associated with low blood levels of CoQ10. Supplementing the diet with CoQ10 helps to reverse the symptoms of periodontal disease. Even applying CoQ10 topically on the gums has shown to significantly improve gum health.[80]

In treating heart disease and cancer, therapeutic doses range from 90-390 mg a day, although positive results have been reported for doses as low as 30 mg per day. There is no official recommended dietary allowance for CoQ10, but 10 to 30 mg a day is generally suggested as a preventative dose. This is far more than you would ordinarily get from diet alone. Red palm oil is one of the richest natural sources of CoQ10. It contains about 45 mg/kg of CoQ10. Adding red palm oil to your diet can help increase your daily intake of this vital nutrient.

PALM STEROLS

Palm oil contains a variety of plant sterols or phytosterols, most notably sitosterol, stigmasterol, and campesterol. Phytosterols are present in small amounts of 350 to 650 parts per million in red palm oil and 100 to 160 parts per million in refined palm oil.

The main focus of interest in plant sterols has been their effect in lowering blood cholesterol. The cholesterol-lowering effect of plant sterols is so powerful that, years ago, before the cholesterol-lowering drugs of today, phytosterol based products were prescribed for people with high blood cholesterol. These products were successful, but not as convenient to take, as the drugs nowadays.

The first studies that showed phytosterols reduced blood cholesterol was in the early 1950s. Dr. Farquhar of Stanford University was a pioneer in this field. He found that LDL (the bad) cholesterol was reduced by 20 percent when subjects with high blood cholesterol consumed 12 to 18 grams of plant sterols each day. Plant sterols act by restraining the absorption of cholesterol in two ways. First they limit the absorption of cholesterol obtained from the diet. Second, they also limit absorption of cholesterol in the intestinal tract.

Recent studies show that intakes of 2-3 grams of phytosterols a day result in LDL cholesterol reductions ranging from 10-15 percent. Some recent studies have shown equal reductions with much smaller daily doses such as 0.7 to 0.8 grams. Thus the amount of phytosterols in foods can have an impact on cholesterol levels.

Although phytosterols have shown promise in lowering cholesterol levels, they have received more attention in the treatment of benign prostatic hyperplasia (enlarged prostate). Phytosterols have been in use in Europe for many years to treat benign prostatic hyperplasia or BPH. A number of studies show reduction of symptoms and increased urine flow after treatment with phytosterols.[81, 82]

A popular herbal treatment for BPH is saw palmetto berries. The active ingredient in saw palmetto berries that make it useful in treating BPH are phytosterols. Saw palmetto is a member of the palm family and the phytosterols in the berries are the same as those found in the fruit of the palm tree and in red palm oil, which is extracted from the fruit.

WHITE PALM OIL
White or refined palm oil is the most common type of palm oil used in the commercial food industry. On food ingredient labels, refined palm oil is listed simply as "palm oil." Unrefined palm oil is generally

Tocopherol, Tocotrienol, and Carotene Content in Corn, Soybean, and Palm Oils (mg/kg)

Substance	Corn Oil	Soybean Oil	Red Palm Oil	White Palm Oil
Alpha-T	126	28	143	97
Gamma-T	446	235	nd	nd
Delta-T	25	145	nd	nd
Total T	597	408	143	97
Alpha-T3	nd	nd	188	161
Gamma-T3	nd	nd	296	203
Delta-T3	nd	nd	81	51
Total T3	nil	nil	565	415
Carotenes	nd	nd	584	nd

Nd=not detected T=tocopherols T3=tocotrienols

Source: Sundram, K., et al. Effect of dietary palm oils on mammary carcinogenesis in female rats induced by 7,12-dimethylbenz(a)anthracene. *Cancer Res* 1989;49:1447-1451.

indicated as "red palm oil" or sometimes "virgin palm oil." Like virgin olive oil, virgin or red palm oil is considered to be a better quality oil because it is less processed and contains a higher nutrient content. Consequently, it is also a bit more expensive.

When red palm oil is refined and transformed into white palm oil, some of its nutrients are removed. With a relatively high saturated fat content and fewer nutrients, some may question whether white palm oil is still good to eat. The answer is "yes." Although red palm oil is nutritionally superior, white palm oil is still a healthy choice.

Carotenes give virgin palm oil its distinctive red color. When palm oil is refined, almost all of the carotenes are removed. Thus the oil becomes a light yellow when liquid or white when solid. Not all of the nutrients are lost however. While some tocopherols and tocotrienols are removed, surprisingly most of them remain. Refined palm oil retains 67 percent of tocopherols, 73 percent of the tocotrienols. So white palm oil is still a good source of vitamin E. White palm oil is chemically stable, resistant to oxidation, and contains the antioxidant power of tocopherols and tocotrienols.

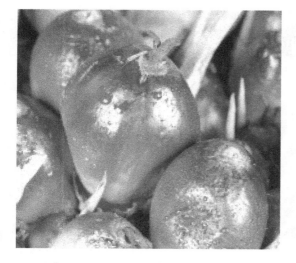

Palm fruit grows in bunches containing a thousand or more individual fruitlets. Each fruitlet is about the size of a small plum. Bunches are harvested about every month. Palm oil is extracted from the flesh of the fruit.

Above is a table comparing the vitamin E and beta-carotene content of soybean oil, corn oil, red palm oil, and white palm oil. Corn oil contains a total of 597 mg/kg of vitamin E, soybean oil 408 mg/kg, red palm oil 708 mg/kg (as well as 584 mg/kg of carotenes), and white palm oil 512 mg/kg. Most of the vitamin E in the two palm oils are the much more potent tocotrienols. Even the refined white palm oil is superior to corn and soybean oils because of its tocotrienol content. In studies where cancer is chemically induced in lab animals, both red and white palm oils block tumor development in comparison to corn and soybean oils.[83]

Vegetable oils provide 60 percent of vitamin E in our diet. Fruits and vegetables contribute another 10 percent. Grains, nuts, and meats supply most of the remaining 30 percent. Animal fats and processed foods contribute a negligible amount. Therefore, the oils in our diet supply us with most of our vitamin E requirements. The best source of vitamin E is palm oil, both white and red.

Chapter 5

Palm Oil and Heart Disease

PALM OIL AND HEART DISEASE

The biggest concern people have about using palm oil is that it contains a high amount of saturated fat. Fifty percent of the oil consists of saturated fat. Saturated fats are supposed to be bad for the heart. So does palm oil cause heart disease? If you believed the advertisements and articles sponsored by the vegetable oil and drug industries and the misguided warnings of the media who blindly criticize *all* saturated fats, you would think so. Despite the many voices speaking out in popular diet books and periodicals that have condemned palm oil, no studies back up this presumption. Why? Because it isn't true. Numerous studies have evaluated the effect that palm oil has on cholesterol levels and other risk factors for heart disease, and the consensus among researchers is that palm oil does not promote heart disease. If anything, it *protects* against it!

So why isn't palm oil given credit as one of the heart friendly vegetable oils? The reason is because of the strong anti-saturated fat sentiment among laypeople, writers, and medical professionals alike and their general lack of knowledge about diet and nutrition. People get most, if not all, of their education on dietary fats and nutrition from newspapers and popular diet books, the authors of which, generally know little or nothing about palm oil. They haven't taken the time to actually read or even research the facts about palm oil. They glean their information from the marketing and promotional literature produced by big business and what previous misinformed authors have written.

73

Few writers of health and diet books actually take the time or effort to read any of the published studies on palm oil. It's not like the information is hidden. It is easily accessible to anyone, especially if you have access to the Internet. PubMed is an Internet database of thousands of studies published by the most prestigious medical and scientific journals in the world. Anybody can access this information and read the studies. I would estimate that 90 percent of the authors who write about diet and health never bother to use this resource or verify the information they write about. It is much easier to rely on previously published works and just rephrase the ideas from other authors. This way old, outdated ideas keep resurfacing in newly published books and periodicals. For this reason, much of the material written about fats and oils is wrong. This is why many people are confused.

Let's look at what the studies actually say about palm oil. I have included references to many of the studies so if you are skeptical about what I say, you can look them up and read them for yourself. The purpose of this book is to uncover the truth, not promote big business, therefore, this information may be totally new to you.

PALM OIL MYTHS

Most people are misinformed and confused about the true nature of palm oil. They think it contains cholesterol or it will raise their blood cholesterol or in some way promote heart disease. Let me put those myths to rest and briefly address the major criticisms palm oil has received over the years.

Myth 1: Pam Oil Contains Cholesterol

One of the biggest misconceptions many people have about palm oil is that because it contains saturated fat, it must also contain cholesterol. Only animal fats contain cholesterol. Palm oil is a vegetable oil and, therefore, contains absolutely no cholesterol.

Like all other unrefined vegetable oils, palm oil, and particularly red palm oil, contains a modest amount of plant sterols which are similar in structure to cholesterol. Plant sterols or phytosterols are not involved in the atherosclerotic process and do not promote heart disease. Plant sterols can, however, lower blood cholesterol. When consumed with cholesterol, competition between the two reduces the amount of cholesterol that is absorbed into the blood stream.[1, 2]

Studies have shown that even moderate amounts of phytosterols added to the diet can lower total cholesterol by 12 percent, LDL cholesterol by 15 percent and improve the cholesterol ratio by 25 percent.[3] That's a significant change! Therefore, the phytosterols in red palm oil can help improve blood cholesterol levels.

Myth 2: Palm Oil is An Artery-Clogging Saturated Fat

The phrase "artery-clogging saturated fat" in reference to tropical oils was coined by The Center for Science in the Public Interest (CSPI), a staunchly anti-saturated fat consumer advocacy organization. The phrase was used to instill fear in the minds of the public against palm and other tropical oils and has been a favorite battle cry of theirs for over two decades. Many other anti-fat zealots have taken up the battle cry and often repeat it in their promotional and educational materials. The problem with this statement is that not only is it untrue, it doesn't even make sense.

Palm oil contains saturated fat, but saturated fat does not clog arteries! At least not like unsaturated fats do. An examination of the fatty acids in arterial plaque reveals that most of the fat that clogs up arteries is *unsaturated*. Seventy-four percent of the fat in arterial plaque is unsaturated.[4] Only oxidized fats become sticky and cling to artery walls. Normal, non-oxidized fats do not. Polyunsaturated fats are very vulnerable to oxidation both in and outside of the body. Monounsaturated fats are also vulnerable but less so. Saturated fats are highly resistant to oxidation and are not easily oxidized.

Fats and cholesterol are transported together throughout the body in the form of lipoproteins. When polyunsaturated fats become oxidized, they generate free radicals that attack and oxidize the other fats and the cholesterol within the lipoprotein. All the fats in the lipoprotein become oxidized. These oxidized lipids are the ones that end up getting stuck to artery walls.

Oxidation causes fats to become hard and sticky. For this reason, soybean oil and other highly polyunsaturated fats are used to make paint, varnish, and ink. Polyunsaturated vegetable oils served as the base for most paints and varnishes until the late 1940s when cheaper synthetic petroleum-based oils came into use. Saturated fats aren't used for this purpose because it is too difficult to oxidize them. Arterial plaque is filled with hardened, sticky unsaturated fats. In truth then, unsaturated fats, and particularly polyunsaturated fats, are the real artery-clogging fats.

Myth 3: Palm Oil Raises Blood Cholesterol

Saturated fats tend to raise blood cholesterol. Polyunsaturated fats tend to lower cholesterol. Monounsaturated fats are more or less neutral. While in general these statements are true, they represent a gross oversimplification.

No oil is 100 percent saturated or polyunsaturated or monounsaturated. All natural fats contain a mixture of all thee types of fatty acids, and the percentage of each varies. A fat is considered saturated if it is predominately composed of saturated fatty acids. Similarly with mono- and polyunsaturated fats. Therefore, every dietary fat will have a different effect on blood cholesterol, depending on its fatty acid profile.

The saturated fatty acids in an oil may raise cholesterol while the polyunsaturated fatty acids lower it. So the ratio of saturated fatty acids to polyunsaturated fatty acids will determine, to some extent, the overall effect the oil will have on blood cholesterol.

This issue is further complicated by the fact that there are many different types of saturated fatty acids just as there are many polyunsaturated and monounsaturated fatty acids and each can have a different effect on cholesterol. For example, there are nine different saturated fatty acids that are relatively common in the human diet.

These saturated fatty acids are found in foods of both animal and plant origin. Soybean oil, for instance, although it contains mostly unsaturated fatty acids, also contains both stearic and palmitic acids. By far the most abundant saturated fats in the diet are stearic and

Saturated Fatty Acids		
Butyric	Capric	Palmitic
Caproic	Lauric	Stearic
Caprylic	Myristic	Arachidic

palmitic acids. What's interesting is that out of the nine saturated fatty acids, only *three* tend to raise blood cholesterol.[5, 6] The rest have either a cholesterol-lowering or a neutral effect. So contrary to popular belief, most saturated fatty acids do not raise blood cholesterol.

The hypercholesterolemic (cholesterol rising) saturated fatty acids are lauric, myristic, and palmitic acids. You will notice that palmitic acid, which is the primary saturated fatty acid in palm oil, is among these. This is where much of the confusion arises. Because palmitic acid tends to increase cholesterol, people assume that any fat that contains palmitic acid is hypercholesterolemic.

To confuse the issue even more, the combination of fatty acids, both saturated and unsaturated, also affects cholesterol response. Palmitic acid is hypercholesterolemic *only* if the diet is also either very high in cholesterol or very low in linoleic acid.[7, 8]

Linoleic acid is the most abundant polyunsaturated fatty acid found in our foods. Soybean, corn, safflower and other polyunsaturated vegetable oils are composed predominately of linoleic acid. Linoleic acid is one of the essential fatty acids (EFA). Low dietary intake of linoleic acid can lead to an essential fatty acid deficiency. Some of the symptoms associated with an essential fatty acid deficiency are raised cholesterol and atherosclerosis.

Studies show that when linoleic acid is provided in the amount that is typically seen in normal diets, palmitic acid does not raise blood cholesterol. Even high levels of palmitic acid in the diet are not hypercholesterolemic if intake of linoleic acid is adequate.[9] However, when linoleic acid is reduced to 3 percent or less, palmitic acid begins to become hypercholesterolemic. So palmitic acid only raises blood cholesterol when there is a deficiency of linoleic acid. The greater the deficiency, the more hypercholesterolemic palmitic acid becomes.

Linoleic acid is so abundant in nature that a deficiency is normally only seen in experimental diets and in cases of malnutrition. Excess consumption of trans fatty acids from hydrogenated oils can also interfere with linoleic acid absorption and contribute to an essential fatty acid deficiency. Trans fatty acids also raise cholesterol so they can have a pronounced negative effect on cholesterol levels.

Researchers can control the cholesterol response in test subjects by adjusting the amount of linoleic acid, trans fatty acids, and cholesterol in experimental diets. If they want the cholesterol in subjects to increase, they can reduce the essential fatty acids to a critical level or increase trans fatty acids or cholesterol. If a researcher wants to show that palm oil or palmitic acid raises cholesterol, he can manipulate the other fats in the diet to accomplish this. Some researchers do this purposely to achieve the results they or their sponsors want. Others do it inadvertently. This is why many studies appear to be contradictory or inconclusive.

Only under certain conditions is palmitic acid hypercholesterolemic. People eating normal diets with adequate nutrients don't have to worry. Keep in mind, palm oil is not pure palmitic acid. It consists of a combination of at least eight different fatty acids. Only 44 percent is palmitic acid. Another 40 percent is oleic acid, the type of monounsaturated fatty acid found in olive oil, which has a neutral effect on cholesterol. It also contains 10 percent linoleic acid, which lowers blood cholesterol. Linoleic acid is naturally present is all grains, vegetables, and meats. So, even if the only fat you use in your diet was palm oil, it would be nearly impossible to develop a deficiency in linoleic acid. Therefore, palm oil would not raise your cholesterol. In studies where adequate linoleic acid was included in diets, palm oil did not raise cholesterol and helped to prevent atherosclerosis.[10-12]

Palm oil, especially red palm oil, contains an abundance of phytonutrients such as phytosterols, tocopherols, and tocotrienols, all of which have a cholesterol lowering effect. Natural non-hydrogenated palm oil when used in a normal diet does not have a negative effect on blood cholesterol. Some studies have shown that it can even *lower* cholesterol.[13]

Myth 4: Many Studies Show Palm Oil Causes Heart Disease

Hardly a week goes by that I don't see in the news or read in a book or on the Internet the warning to avoid tropical oils because they are high in saturated fat and lead to heart disease. Even government health guidelines recommend avoiding palm oil. With so many warnings from so many places, you would think there must be an overwhelming amount of evidence supporting the position that palm oil causes heart disease.

The diet-heart disease connection has been studied meticulously for over 60 years. Surely in that amount of time, enough evidence has mounted to definitively prove the connection between palm oil and heart

78

disease. Indeed, thousands of studies have been published on palm oil, palmitic acid, saturated fats, and related topics. Yet, despite the mountain of research, no studies prove that palm oil causes heart disease. There are studies that allude to it by lumping palm oil in with other saturated fats or trans fats or expounding on the cholesterol rising effect of palmitic acid. But as we have seen in Myth 3, palmitic acid is only hypercholesterolemic under certain conditions. Palm oil when used as a part of a normal diet does not raise cholesterol and some studies show it even lowers it.

There is no credible evidence whatsoever that palm oil contributes in any way to the development of heart disease. However, there are numerous studies that demonstrate that palm oil is harmless and may even help protect against heart disease.

Myth 5: People Who Eat Palm Oil Die From Heart Disease

If palm oil were the deadly artery-clogging saturated fat the media has made it out to be, heart disease would be rampant in those populations around the world which eat large amounts of it. These people should have high heart attack and stroke rates. However, when you examine the health statistics of countries like Malaysia, Indonesia, and West Africa where palm oil consumption is relatively high, you find that heart disease is extremely low compared to the United States, Europe, Australia and other countries in the world that consume little palm oil.

In southwestern Nigeria palm oil is used almost exclusively. People have a relatively high consumption of saturated fat and in general consume a substantial amount of meat, eggs, and milk. Total fat consumption is 37 percent.[14] This is considered very high. The American Heart Association recommends that we limit our total fat consumption to 30 percent of calories with the desired range of around 20-25 percent. Despite the fact that these Nigerians eat far more fat than that and the majority of it is saturated fat, they have a very low incidence of heart disease. In fact, in Nigeria coronary heart disease is considered rare.[15]

In a study of hospital admissions from 1975 to 1976 at the Ahmadu Bello University Teaching Hospital in Kaduna, Nigeria there was not a single case of coronary heart disease reported among native Nigerians.[16] There were, however, cases among non-Africans. The only cases of heart disease reported among the Nigerian population were caused by infections or malnutrition.

Studies involving urbanized Nigerians who work and live in an environment similar to many Americans and Europeans show much better blood cholesterol values.[17] Both urbanized and rural Nigerians have a low incidence of coronary heart disease.

WHAT IS HEART DISEASE?

In order to really understand the heart disease issue in relationship to palm oil, you need to know what heart disease is. Heart disease is a generalized term referring to any disease affecting the heart or circulatory system. The term is most commonly used to describe an advanced stage of atherosclerosis which leads to heart attacks and strokes.

Atherosclerosis or hardening of the arteries is characterized by the formation of plaque in the arteries. If you asked most people what causes atherosclerosis, they would probably tell you it was from too much cholesterol in the blood. But cholesterol doesn't simply come dancing merrily down the artery and suddenly decide to stick somewhere. In fact, cholesterol isn't even necessary for atherosclerosis or the formation of plaque. The body uses cholesterol to patch up and repair injuries to the arterial wall. Contrary to popular belief, the principle component of arterial plaque is not cholesterol but protein, mainly in the form of scar tissue. Some atherosclerotic arteries actually contain little or no cholesterol.

In the currently accepted response-to-injury hypothesis of atherosclerosis, plaque initially develops as a result of an injury to the inner lining of the arterial wall. The injury can be the result of a number of factors such as damage from toxins, free radicals, viruses, or bacteria. If the cause of the injury is not removed, further damage may result, and as long as irritation and inflammation persist, scar tissue continues to develop.

When blood-clotting proteins (platelets) encounter an injury, they become sticky and adhere to each other and to the damaged tissue, acting somewhat like a bandage to facilitate healing. This is how blood clots are formed. Injury from any source triggers platelets to clump together, or clot, and arterial cells to release protein growth factors that stimulate growth of the muscle cells within the artery walls. A complex

80

mixture of scar tissue, platelets, calcium, cholesterol, and triglycerides is incorporated into the site to patch up the fissure and heal the injury. This mass of fibrous tissue, not cholesterol, forms the principle material in plaque. The calcium deposits in the plaque cause the hardening, which is characteristic of atherosclerosis.

Contrary to popular belief, plaque isn't simply plastered along the inside of the artery canal like it was mud in a garden hose. It grows inside the artery wall, becoming part of the artery wall itself. Arterial walls are surrounded by a layer of strong circular muscles that prevent the plaque from expanding outward. As the plaque grows, it can't expand outward, so it grows inward, narrowing the artery opening and limiting blood flow.

Platelets gather at the site of injury to form blood clots. If the injury persists or if the blood is prone to clotting, clots may continue to grow to the point that they completely block the flow of blood in the artery. An artery already narrowed by plaque can easily be blocked by blood clots.

The arteries transport oxygen enriched blood throughout the body. Every cell, every tissue, and every organ requires a constant supply of oxygen. Without oxygen, tissues and organs quickly suffocate and die. If the coronary artery, which feeds the heart, is blocked, the result is a heart attack. If the carotid artery, which goes to the brain, is blocked the result is a stroke.

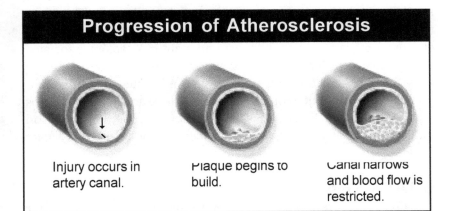

Progression of Atherosclerosis

Injury occurs in artery canal.

Plaque begins to build.

Canal narrows and blood flow is restricted.

Heart disease is a generalized term used most often to describe an advanced stage of atherosclerosis which can lead to a heart attack or stroke. You often hear it referred to as *coronary heart disease*, meaning the coronary arteries which deliver blood and oxygen to the heart become blocked by plaque, which may eventually lead to a heart attack.

There are many forms of heart disease. When people speak of heart disease they are usually referring to coronary heart disease.

PALM OIL FIGHTS HEART DISEASE

Although many factors are undoubtedly involved in heart disease, the exact cause is still unknown. In the search for a cause, researchers have assembled a list of risk factors associated with heart disease. Risk factors do not necessarily cause heart disease, but are conditions which often occur in conjunction with it. For instance, being male is a known risk factor. More men die of heart disease than women. However, being a male does not cause heart disease. Age is another risk factor. Again, age does not cause heart disease, but the older you are, the greater your risk of developing heart disease.

Some risk factors like age, gender, and heredity we have no control over. Most risk factors, however, can be influenced by decisions we make. Smoking is one of these. You can reduce your risk by not smoking. Diet and lifestyle also influence risk.

The more risk factors a person has, the higher the likelihood he or she will experience a heart attack. The opposite is also true. Therefore, those people who have the fewest risk factors are the least likely to encounter a heart attack. The most important risk factors associated with heart disease that you can influence by dietary means are oxidative stress, blood cholesterol levels, hypertension, inflammation, and diabetes. Palm oil as it turns out, reduces each one of these and, therefore, helps *lower* your risk of heart disease. Let's take a look at how palm oil influences each of these risk factors. Diabetes will be covered in Chapter 7.

Oxidative Stress

Oxidative stress is one of the most significant risk factors for atherosclerosis and heart disease. While some risk factors show only an association with heart disease, oxidative stress takes an active part in the process.

An examination of the fats and cholesterol in arterial plaque reveals that they are not ordinary fats, but chemically altered oxidized fats. Oxidized fats are damaged or rancid fats that spawn destructive free radicals. All of the fats that collect in arterial plaque are oxidized. Only oxidized fats are attracted to and adhere to artery walls.

Unsaturated fats and cholesterol in our bodies are the most vulnerable to oxidation. They are easily oxidized by free radicals and, in turn, create more free radicals. Heating polyunsaturated oils, as is typically done in cooking, oxidizes fats. Pollution, chemicals, as well as natural processes in the body also contribute to the formation of free radicals which attack cholesterol and other fats in our bodies. These are the fats that collect in artery walls.

The antioxidant defense system of the body fights a never ending battle defending against free radicals. Oxidative stress occurs when our antioxidant defenders are overwhelmed by excessive free radicals. In this situation more fats are oxidized and, therefore, more oxidized fat is available to be incorporated into arterial plaque. Free radicals may also contribute to inflammation in the arteries which promotes the atherosclerotic process.

Oxidative stress is influenced to a great extent by the foods we eat. Heat damaged vegetable oils and nutrient deficient convenience foods are two of the biggest contributors. Replacing vegetable oils you may ordinarily use in cooking with palm oil can have a big influence on your antioxidant status and oxidative stress. Palm oil is composed of 90 percent saturated and monounsaturated fatty acids. These fats are far more stable than polyunsaturated fats and resist oxidation. Saturated fats are extremely resistant to oxidation. This makes palm oil a safer oil to use in cooking and food preparation.

Red palm oil is loaded with protective antioxidants—alpha-tocopherol, alpha-tocotrienol, gamma-tocotrienol, delta-tocotrienol, alpha-carotene, beta-carotene, gamma-carotene, lycopene, squalene, CoQ10, and others, the most powerful of the bunch being the tocotrienols.

Antioxidants slow or stop the progression of atherosclerosis by blocking the process that oxidizes unsaturated fats and cholesterol. Studies show that low antioxidant status in individuals increases incidence of heart disease.[18, 19] Adding antioxidants into the diet lowers the amount of oxidized fat and cholesterol in the bloodstream and thus reduces atherosclerosis.[20-23]

Population studies have shown that the more antioxidants consumed, the lower the risk of heart disease.[24] In the Nurses Health Study, involving over 887,000 women, a 41 percent reduction in risk of heart disease was reported among nurses who had taken vitamin E for more than two years.[25] The average intake in the lowest-risk group was 200 IU. In the Health Professionals Follow-Up Study involving almost 40,000 men, researchers found men who had taken vitamin E for more than two years had a 37 percent lower risk of heart disease compared to men who had not taken supplements.[26]

In the Cambridge Heart Antioxidant Study, 1000 men with heart problems were given either 400 or 800 IU of vitamin E. After 18 months, the risk of heart attack was reduced by 75 percent in the group receiving supplements.[27]

Because of its high antioxidant content, palm oil protects the heart and arteries from lipid peroxidation.[28] Palm oil helps maintain antioxidant status even when the antioxidant system is severely challenged.[29] Therefore, palm oil is antiatherogenic. In other words, it helps prevent the formation of plaque in arteries.[30]

Cholesterol

The risk factor most widely associated with heart disease in the minds of the public is blood cholesterol. Earlier in this chapter we showed that palm oil in normal diets does not have an adverse effect on cholesterol levels. Here we will see that not only is palm oil not harmful, but it improves those cholesterol values which are most closely associated with heart disease prevention.

Palm oil is the richest dietary source of vitamin E. It is especially rich in tocotrienols. For this reason, vitamin E rich red palm oil has been encapsulated for use as a dietary supplement. This supplement supplies a natural source of mixed tocopherols and tocotrienols as well as a mixture of carotenes and other phytonutrients. A 300 mg capsule of red palm oil contains 18 mg of tocopherols and 42 mg of tocotrienols. Palm oil capsules are convenient to use in studies.

Tocopherols and tocotrienols exert positive effects on cholesterols values. For instance, in one study researchers at the University of Illinois College of Medicine demonstrated a 10 percent decrease in total

84

What Do Doctors Do to Prevent Heart Attacks?

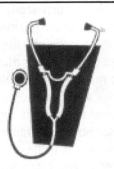

What do cardiologists—medical doctors who specialize in treating heart and related illnesses—do for themselves to prevent heart disease? Most of them take antioxidant vitamins.

A survey among members of the American Academy of Cardiology revealed that 54% routinely take antioxidants. The most common dosages: 400 IU of vitamin E, 500 mg of vitamin C, and 20,000 IU of beta-carotene. Why are so many cardiologists taking antioxidant vitamins? Studies are showing promising results.

A population-based study conducted in Canada with 2,313 men demonstrated vitamin supplement use was associated with a 69 percent reduced risk of death due to coronary artery disease and a 47% reduced risk for a non-fatal heart attack. (*Canadian Journal of Cardiology* 1996;12:930)

In the Cambridge Antioxidant Heart Study, 2,002 patients with coronary artery disease were given either vitamin E or a placebo for 510 days. Vitamin E supplementation reduced the number of patients experiencing a heart attack by an impressive 77 percent (*Lancet* 1996, 347:781).

In two major studies involving a total of nearly one million men and women an average of 40 percent reduction in risk of heart disease was reported after taking vitamin E for more than two years. (*New England Journal of Medicine* 1993;328:1444-1449 and 1450-1456.)

More cardiologists take vitamins than low-dose aspirin—the standard preventive treatment for heart disease. Aspirin works by thinning the blood. Most cardiologists, however, believe that preventing oxidative damage to the arteries to be a better solution to the problem—they must or they wouldn't take the vitamins themselves.

Source: Mehta, J. 1997. Intake of antioxidants among American cardiologists. *Am J Cardiol* 79:1558.

cholesterol in 36 hypercholesterolemic (high cholesterol) subjects given the palm oil capsule for four weeks. A follow-up study of 16 subjects resulted in a 13 percent lowering of cholesterol.[31, 32]

In another study involving 31 subjects cholesterol levels were evaluated at the beginning of the study and again 30 days later. Subjects took one palm oil capsule every day for the 30 days. No other changes were made to their diets. They continued to eat whatever they desired. The results showed that the palm oil lowered both total cholesterol and LDL (bad) cholesterol in *all* the volunteers. The magnitude of reduction of total cholesterol ranged from 5 to 35.9 percent and the reduction of LDL cholesterol ranged from 0.9 to 37 percent. What was even more important was the effect the palm oil had on the cholesterol ratio. The cholesterol ratio was reduced in 78 percent of the subjects, demonstrating a highly significant and favorable response to palm oil supplementation.[33]

The cholesterol ratio is superior to total cholesterol as an indicator of heart disease risk.[34] HDL cholesterol is believed to protect against heart disease while LDL cholesterol is believed to promote it. The amount of each influences heart disease risk. A measurement of total cholesterol is essentially worthless because you don't know how much of each makes up the total. This is why half of all those people who die of heart attacks have normal to below normal total cholesterol levels. The cholesterol ratio (total cholesterol/HDL cholesterol) is a far better indicator of heart disease risk. Both red and white palm oils tend to raise HDL cholesterol and thus improve the cholesterol ratio.

In addition to HDL and LDL cholesterol, other types of cholesterol influence heart disease risk. LDL cholesterol is often combined with another compound known as apolipoprotein B (apo B). Apo B increases the transport capacity of low-density cholesterol in the bloodstream and, therefore, is believed to increase the ability of cholesterol to be deposited on artery walls. Many researchers believe it is a better indicator of heart disease risk than LDL cholesterol alone. Patients with arterial plaque often show a high percentage of apo B in their blood, so reducing apo B is believed to reduce risk of heart disease. Studies indicate that palm oil tends to reduce the concentration of apolipoprotein B and, therefore, reduce risk of heart disease.[35]

In a study carried out in Holland, researchers evaluated the effect of replacing the usual sources of fat in the Dutch diet by palm oil. The following significant results were obtained:

1. No effect on plasma total cholesterol
2. An 11 percent increase in HDL cholesterol
3. A 8 percent decrease in LDL cholesterol
4. An 9 percent decrease in triglycerides
5. An increase in plasma apolipoprotein A1 (a type of HDL) and decrease in apolipoprotein B (apo B), both positive changes.

The researchers concluded that the changes demonstrate the heart protective nature of the palm oil.[36]

Another type of LDL cholesterol is lipoprotein(a) or Lp(a). It is similar in structure to LDL but with the addition of another compound known as apolipoprotein(a). Apolipoprotein(a) is an adhesive protein that encourages sticking to artery walls. Lp(a) has been identified as a separate and distinct risk factor for heart disease. Lp(a) is associated with ten times the risk of elevated LDL, which on its own lacks the sticky properties of apolipoprotein(a). Studies indicate that Lp(a) and LDL cholesterol work synergistically together in promoting atherosclerosis and heart disease. Some researchers believe that Lp(a) is the single most important lipid in assessing a person's true risk of developing heart disease.

Lowering Lp(a) levels is correlated with a reduced risk of heart disease.[37] Cholesterol-lowering drugs have been ineffective in lowering Lp(a) levels. While genetics may predispose some people to have elevated Lp(a), it is also influenced by diet. Trans fats increase Lp(a) while vegetables, fruits, and nuts reduce it.[38, 39] Several studies have shown palm oil to be effective in reducing lipoprotein(a) in blood, thus reducing risk of heart disease.[40-43]

While palm oil doesn't have much affect on total cholesterol, it has a positive effect on HDL cholesterol, the cholesterol ratio, apo B, and Lp(a) all of which indicate its protective nature against heart disease.

Hypertension

Researchers have long associated hypertension or high blood pressure with an increased risk of atherosclerosis. High blood pressure appears to be both a major cause and a consequence of atherosclerosis. High blood pressure puts undue stress on artery walls which can cause minute tears within the lining of the walls, leading to the sequence of events that causes the build up of plaque. In turn, atherosclerotic arteries which are narrowed with plaque cause blood pressure to build as the heart is forced to pump the same volume of blood through smaller passageways.

One of the primary factors that affect blood pressure is the stickiness of the blood. The blood contains special proteins called platelets. When a blood vessel is injured these platelets are activated and become sticky, causing blood cells to clump together to form clots at the injury site. The clots adhere to the injured tissues to prevent blood loss and to facilitate healing. Chronic inflammation, infections, free radicals, and other factors activate platelet stickiness, causing blood cells to stick to one another. As they do, the blood becomes "thicker" or more viscous. The heart has to work harder to pump the blood through the arteries, and pressure increases, thus setting into motion the process that leads to atherosclerosis.

Vitamin E acts as a blood thinner by reducing platelet activation and blood pressure.[44, 45] Animal and human studies have shown that vitamin E rich palm oil does the same thing. Palm oil reduces platelet stickiness, blood clot formation, and atherosclerosis.[46-50]

Another factor that increases blood pressure is oxidative stress. Oxidative stress promotes inflammation and injury that activates platelets. As discussed earlier, palm oil can reduce oxidative stress. In so doing, elevated blood pressure is also lowered.[51, 52]

Artery walls are elastic and can expand and contract as conditions dictate. For instance, as the heart contracts and pumps blood through the blood vessels, the arteries expand to allow the blood to flow through easily. Between beats, as the heart relaxes, the arteries contract in order to maintain pressure and facilitate blood flow. Also during times of physical activity, the arteries dilate to increase blood flow in order to deliver an increased amount of oxygen to working muscles.

Irritation to the layer of cells along the inside of the artery wall causes inflammation and swelling. Swelling narrows the artery passageway, restricting blood flow, which in turn increases blood pressure.

People with hypertension are advised to reduce salt intake because it can cause artery walls to swell. Excess salt in the diet irritates artery walls, which in turn causes the formation of free radicals, promotes

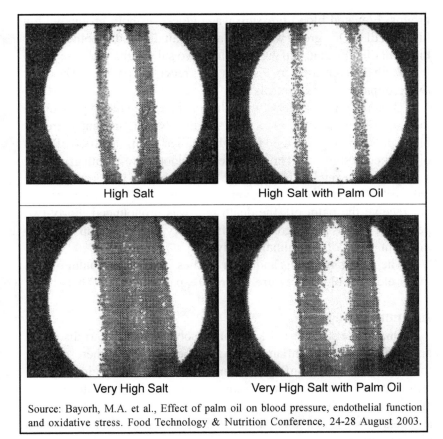

| High Salt | High Salt with Palm Oil |
| Very High Salt | Very High Salt with Palm Oil |

Source: Bayorh, M.A. et al., Effect of palm oil on blood pressure, endothelial function and oxidative stress. Food Technology & Nutrition Conference, 24-28 August 2003.

Digitized images showing density changes in the thickness and diameter of artery walls in rats with salt-induced hypertension. Notice how both the high and very high salt diets have decreased the diameter of the arteries and narrowed the passageways restricting blood flow. In the palm oil fed rats, the arteries remained wider, allowing greater blood flow.

swelling, and increases blood pressure. Researchers can induce high blood pressure in animals by feeding them high salt diets. In salt sensitive animals, elevated blood pressure can be reduced by giving them antioxidants.[53]

The antioxidants in palm oil can lower salt-induced hypertension. In one study, for instance, salt-sensitive rats were divided into two groups. Elevated blood pressure was induced in both groups with a high salt diet. One group was given a high salt diet and the other a very high salt diet. Each group was split into two subgroups with one group from both the high and very high salt diets receiving palm oil. The other two groups served as controls.

Both the high and very high salt diets increased blood pressure in the rats. Rats given the very high salt diet had significantly greater blood pressure than those on the high salt diet. Administration of palm oil resulted in significant improvement of blood flow in both groups.

All of the rats in the high salt group whether they received the palm oil or not survived. However, in the very high salt group that did not receive the palm oil, the death rate was pronounced. Forty-two percent of the rats in this group died. In the very high salt group receiving the palm oil *all* of the animals survived.[54]

The results from this and other studies indicate that palm oil can lower elevated blood pressure. Therefore, palm oil is heart healthy.

Inflammation

One of the strongest risk factors associated with heart disease is arterial inflammation. Inflammation must be present for atherosclerosis to develop. Chronic inflammation encourages blood clotting and stimulates the formation of scar tissue that is characteristic of atherosclerosis. The relationship between chronic arterial inflammation and heart disease is a much better indicator of heart disease risk than high cholesterol.

The degree of arterial inflammation can be determined by measuring a substance in the blood called C-reactive protein (CRP). Dr. Paul Ridker of Brigham and Women's Hospital in Boston evaluated blood samples from more than 28,000 healthy nurses. Those with the highest levels of C-reactive protein had more than four times the risk of having heart trouble. He says, "We were able to find that the C-reactive protein is a stronger predictor of risk than were the regular cholesterol levels, and that's very important because almost half of all heart attacks occur among people who have normal cholesterol levels."[55]

Inflammation of the arteries may explain heart disease in people without other known risk factors—people with normal cholesterol and low blood pressure who are non-diabetic and in good physical shape.

These patients make up a third of all heart attack cases. Researchers have known for years that other factors must be involved in coronary artery disease.

Interleukin-6 is a substance produced by our cells that stimulates inflammation and tells the liver to make C-reactive protein. The overproduction of interleukin-6 has been implicated in many inflammatory health problems including rheumatoid arthritis, Crohn's disease, and heart disease. Consequently, researchers are seeking ways to moderate interleukin-6 production.

Vitamin E is known to reduce inflammation, in part by reducing interleukin-6 production.[56] Tocotrienols from palm oil are the most effective. Tocotrienols temper the production of interleukin-6 and thus ease inflammation.[57]

Dietary supplementation with vitamin E alone reduces inflammation. Combining CoQ10 with vitamin E significantly enhances the anti-inflammatory effects of vitamin E.[58]

Palm oil, which contains both tocotrienols and CoQ10, also possesses anti-inflammatory effects. When palm oil is used in place of polyunsaturated oils in the diet, it reduces chronic inflammation.[59] In one study 38 male volunteers consumed either a diet containing palm oil or one without palm oil (control diet). Each diet lasted 6 weeks. Palm oil was shown to reduce proinflammatory cytokines (including interleukin-6) which promotes inflammation within blood vessels. The residual anti-inflammatory effect of the palm oil lasted more than 9 weeks after the 6 week testing period. Thus it appears that palm oil has a direct moderating effect on inflammation that reduces risk of atherosclerosis.

PALM OIL PROTECTS YOUR HEART

Palm oil is emerging as a premiere heart healthy food. It is loaded with heart protective antioxidants and nutrients that are not found in as great abundance in other foods. Studies are continually being published demonstrating the heart protective nature of this oil.

As noted earlier in this chapter, palm oil does not contribute in any way to the development of heart disease, even though it contains a relatively high percentage of saturated fat. Palm oil, however, isn't just an innocent bystander when it comes to heart health. It takes an active role in protecting the heart and arteries from the conditions that lead to heart attacks and stokes.

Palm oil is loaded with heart protective nutrients such as tocotrienols, alpha- and beta-carotene, and CoQ10. As you have seen in this chapter, palm oil has a beneficial effect on the most important risk factors associated with heart disease. Each one of these risk factors is reduced with the use of palm oil, thus lowering your chances of experiencing a heart attack or stroke.

What palm oil does is truly amazing. It protects the heart from a variety of harmful conditions. In studies where researchers purposely induce heart attacks in lab animals by cutting off blood flow to the heart, palm oil protects the heart, minimizes the injury, and speeds recovery.[60-62] Does a substance that protects the heart from heart attacks cause them? Obviously not. These studies clearly demonstrate the protective nature of the oil.

Studies have shown that the tocotrienols in palm oil actively remove plaque build up in arteries and, therefore, *reverses the progression of atherosclerosis.*[62-65] This has been demonstrated in both animals and humans.

In one study, for instance, 50 subjects were divided into two equal groups. All the participants had been diagnosed with atherosclerosis. One group was given tocotrienol rich palm oil. The other group served as the control. The degree of atherosclerosis was monitored using ultrasound scans over an 18 month period. In the group receiving palm oil, atherosclerosis was halted in 23 of the 25 subjects. In 7 of these subjects atherosclerosis was not only stopped but regressed. In comparison, none of those in the control group showed any improvement, in fact, the condition in 10 worsened.

Cholesterol levels in both groups remained essentially the same. So the regression in arterial plaque was not due to a lowering of cholesterol levels. Although many factors may have been involved, the authors attributed the antioxidant effects of vitamin E in the palm oil as a primary factor.

No other dietary oil has shown to reverse atherosclerosis like palm oil. Therefore, palm oil protects against heart disease better than soybean oil, sunflower oil, corn oil, and all the other so-called "heart friendly" polyunsaturated fats. Even though these fats may have a greater effect on lowering total cholesterol, they do *not* stop or reverse atherosclerosis. Palm oil, therefore, can be of benefit in both preventing and in treating heart disease.

The real proof that shows whether palm oil is good for the heart is what it does in real life outside of laboratories, controlled studies, and contrived diets. How does palm oil affect people who use it every day as a major source of fat in their diet. This is how the oil would be used by you and me on a practical level as a part of normal diet. Is it still heart friendly? Will it still protect the heart and arteries? The answer is a resounding "yes." Those populations who consume palm oil as a part of their everyday diet have a remarkably low rate of heart disease. Does this not validate what the studies have demonstrated?

If you want to avoid becoming a casualty of heart disease, one of the things you should start doing right now is to incorporate palm oil into your daily diet.

Beware of the Critics

When you look at all the evidence supporting the heart friendly nature of palm oil, it is surprising that it has been misrepresented for so long.

Despite the studies demonstrating the health benefits of palm oil, there are still people who criticize it in ignorance. Anyone who says that palm oil causes or promotes heart disease obviously has never taken the time to investigate the subject. Because of people like this, you will continue to read and hear negative comments about palm oil in the news and in books and magazines for some time to come. Some of these people will be respected physicians or best-selling authors. Your own doctor may be behind the times on this one as well. If you tell your doctor you are using palm oil, the reaction you receive may be one of disdain, and you may be strongly urged to stop using it. Don't let such comments trouble you. After reading this book you know far more about palm oil, and probably fats in general, than most physicians.

If you ask critics why they say not to use palm oil, their response will be: "Because it's a saturated fat," as if that in itself is enough proof. But blindly labeling palm oil an "artery clogging" saturated fat simply out of prejudice is irresponsible and reflects poor judgment. After reading this book, you know better.

Chapter 6

Fighting Cancer with Palm Oil

Cancer is second only to heart disease as the leading cause of death in the United States, Canada, Australia, and most of Europe. It is the fifth leading cause of death worldwide. Ten million new cases are diagnosed each year. Despite spending billions of dollars in the war against cancer, the number of cases continues to increase year after year.

Cancer knows no age boundaries; it affects the young as well as the old, although risk increases with age. If you live in North America or Europe you have about a 1 in 3 chance of getting cancer sometime in your lifetime.

Regardless of your age or where you live, you are exposed to cancer every day. Cancerous cells form in our bodies all the time. The reason we don't all come down with cancer is that our immune system wages a constant battle with anything that poses a potential danger, this includes cancerous cells. Anticancer nutrients in our foods also aid the immune system in keeping cancer at bay. A healthy, well nourished body, therefore, is less likely to develop cancer.

Most people recognize cancer as an abnormal growth of tissue. What causes it? Many factors can be involved, including lifestyle choices, poor diet, environmental toxins, radiation, etc. Whatever the cause, the result is an abnormal and unrestrained growth of cells in a particular part of the body. Growths or tumors most commonly develop in major organs, such as the lungs, breasts, intestines, skin, or stomach.

Cancer begins when a mutation occurs in a cell's DNA, which causes it to grow and multiply out of control. Once a cell is transformed, the change is passed on to all offspring cells. Usually the abnormal cells show a lack of differentiation—that is, they no longer perform the specialized task of the cells of their parent tissue. Nerve cells that become cancerous lose the ability to relay messages; pancreas cells lose the ability to make digestive enzymes and hormones; kidney cells lose the ability to filter toxins from the blood, and so on. Cancer cells form a useless mass of tissue. They, in effect, become parasites, contributing nothing to their host tissue but continue to consume nutrients. These abnormal cells grow at an accelerated rate in a random, disorderly way. As the cells multiply, they spread and infiltrate surrounding tissues, eventually interfering with the function of the affected organs.

The word *cancer* is Latin for crab. It is believed that the term was used to describe the shape of a tumorous mass with veins of cancerous tissues extending from the body, looking somewhat like the body of a crab with long legs.

Cancer can spread from one location to practically any part of the body. Cells from the body of the tumor may migrate by way of the blood steam to other parts of the body where they metastasize or form new, satellite tumors that grow independently.

The rate of growth varies, but years may pass before a tumor becomes large enough to cause any noticeable symptoms. Current estimates suggest that some cancers of the lung and breast have been present for more than five years before they become noticeable. Even before symptoms become evident, metastases may already have spread far beyond the primary site of origin.

The most common treatment for most cancers is surgery. Because small, undetectable metastases often remain in the body after an operation, surgery is often combined with radiation and chemotherapy. Surgery is only useful against localized tumors that can be identified and physically removed. Radiation and chemotherapy can influence cancerous cells regardless of their size or where they are in the body.

These treatments, however, can have serious consequences. Surgery often leaves a patient crippled or disfigured. Chemotherapy and radiation are accompanied by severe side effects because many normal cells are killed along with the cancerous cells.

Alternative therapies focus on enhancing the immune system and utilizing a variety of relatively harmless treatments, including the use of cancer protective foods. Many substances found in plants posses immune building and anticancer properties that can be helpful in preventing and treating cancer without the deleterious effects associated with conventional cancer treatments. Palm oil is one of these natural, cancer fighting foods.

PALM OIL FIGHTS CANCER

Fruits and vegetables are rich sources of anticancer nutrients such as vitamin E and carotenes. Many of these nutrients act as antioxidants, which block the processes that initiate cancer development.[1] Red palm oil is especially beneficial in this respect because it provides a rich source of palmetic acid, squalene, carotenes, tocopherols, and tocotrienols, all of which function as protective antioxidants. Palm oil contains the richest natural source of two very powerful cancer fighting nutrients—tocotrienols and gamma-carotene—making it a potent cancer fighting food.

The anticancer power of red palm oil and its individual components is amply documented in medical studies.[2] Researchers have access to all of the major studies being published throughout the world through PubMed. A search on PubMed reveals over 14,000 published studies involving palm oil or its individual components and its effect on cancer. Fourteen thousand studies is a huge amount of research. In recent years the emphasis has been on breast cancer for which palm oil holds much promise.[3-10]

Studies show palm oil or its components are effective against many forms of cancer including skin cancer,[11-16] liver and lung cancer,[17-21] stomach and pancreatic cancers,[22, 23] colorectal cancer,[24-26] prostate cancer,[27] and various other cancers.[28] It's only shortcoming, perhaps, is that it has not been proven as effective against leukemia as it has with these other forms of cancer. But even then, palm oil is completely harmless and has so many other benefits it would be useful for overall health and to strengthen the immune system.

Because of the research, palm oil or tocotrienol-rich fractions/ extracts of palm oil are being recommended as therapeutic treatments against various forms of cancer.

THE SECRET BEHIND PALM OIL

Palm oil's most studied and most recognized benefit is its cancer fighting ability. What is it about palm oil that makes it so useful in this respect? It's not any one thing, but a combination of many factors. Palm oil is composed of several cancer fighting substances which work together synergistically to give the oil its overall effect. Most of the knowledge we have regarding the health aspects of palm oil come from the study of its individual parts. Let's take a look at what researchers have learned about these substances.

Antioxidants

Free-radical damage to DNA has been identified as a, if not the primary, cause of most cancers. Free radicals can be generated in a number of ways by air pollution (e.g., smog, tobacco smoke, etc.), food additives, ionizing radiation (e.g., UV radiation from the sun, X rays, radiation therapy, etc.), environmental and industrial toxins, and even from normal oxidative processes that occur in the body every day.

Free radicals are a normal part of daily living, against which the body has defense mechanisms to protect us from the destruction action of these harmful molecules. Antioxidant enzymes and nutrients in our bodies block or stop the oxidizing reactions that create free radicals. A problem occurs when free-radical formation exceeds the body's ability to keep them under control. This can happen when we are exposed to excessive amounts of free-radical generating influences or when our antioxidant resources are hindered.

Excessive exposure to carcinogenic substances such as industrial chemicals, flavor enhancers, artificial sweeteners, food dyes, molds, viruses, rancid or heat damaged polyunsaturated oils, and the like can overwhelm your antioxidant defense system. Likewise, a poor diet lacking adequate fresh fruits, vegetables, and whole grains won't supply the nutrients needed to replenish antioxidant reserves. It is estimated that environmental factors and lifestyle and dietary choices initiate at lest 80 percent of all cancers.[29]

Even if you are exposed to a heavy amount of carcinogens in your everyday environment, if you eat the right types of foods, your body will have the protection it needs. Palm oil is one of these cancer protective foods. Palm oil with its high saturated and monounsaturated fat content is very stable chemically and does not promote lipid peroxidation. The stability of palm oil helps block free-radical generation and preserve the body's antioxidant defenses.[30]

Palm oil, especially red palm oil, also contains a rich variety of antioxidants. Antioxidants have been shown to decrease the incidence of cancer by arresting the oxidative processes that give rise to cancer causing free radicals.[31] Palm oil provides one of the highest natural sources of dietary antioxidants. It is, in essence, an antioxidant or free-radical blocking powerhouse. Few foods can compare to it in this respect.

The antioxidants, primarily the vitamin E and carotenes, in palm oil possess very potent anticancer properties that provide protection against cancer even beyond their antioxidant effects.[32]

Cancer and Palm Oil Carotenes

Researchers have been aware of the anticancer properties of carotenes and particularly beta-carotene for many years.[33, 34] Studies show that dietary supplementation of beta-carotene and vitamin A inhibits the development of several chemically induced cancers in laboratory animals.[35-37] Beta-carotene is the most extensively studied of the carotenes because it was believed to be the most biologically active with the most potent anticancer properties. Although many studies have shown a strong anticancer effect for beta-carotene, some studies have not. In fact, a few studies even showed an increased risk of cancer. This inconsistency has baffled researchers.

One of the primary studies to question the usefulness of beta-carotene was conducted in Finland. In this study 29,133 male smokers were involved. To the surprise of the researchers, they found that the risk of cancer actually *increased* in smokers who supplemented their diets with beta-carotene.[38] As a result, many physicians began questioning the previous recommendation of taking beta-carotene and began to warn patients against it. Some doctors are now discouraging the use of beta-carotene for this reason.

Numerous studies performed earlier had already shown beta-carotene to be of benefit against cancer. So, why the discrepancy? The answer is simple. In those studies where benefits were seen, the subjects ate whole foods or supplements from natural sources. In the studies where little benefit was shown, the subjects consumed dietary supplements. The supplements contained synthetic beta-carotene, not the type normally found in the diet. Naturally derived beta-carotene is always associated with a mix of other carotenoids. Synthetic beta-carotene is pure. Pure beta-carotene can be converted into vitamin A and appears to be effective against vitamin A deficiency, but to fight cancer, a mixture of carotenoids appears to be necessary. The cancer fighting effects attributed to beta-carotene in earlier studies may actually be the result of a synergistic mixture of beta-carotene with other naturally occurring carotenoids.

Another carotenoid, alpha-carotene, has been shown to possess more potent anticancer properties than beta-carotene and the two of them together work synergistically so that the combination of both is more effective than either one alone.[39] A mixture of alpha-carotene and beta-carotene with other carotenes provides the greatest anticancer effect.

Red palm oil contains a mixture of carotenes, including alpha-carotene and lycopene, which have proven to possess potent anticancer properties. Studies using palm oil containing mixed carotenes have been shown to inhibit the growth of skin, stomach, pancreas, liver, lung, breast, and other cancers.[40-45]

It is of interest to note that the Finish study showed an increase in lung cancer among smokers who took beta-carotene supplements. However, in other studies using a mix of natural carotenes derived from palm oil, lung cancer was reduced. While beta-carotene supplements may not provide protection from cancer, palm oil with mixed carotenes does.

Cancer and Tocotrienols

The form of vitamin E most commonly found in our foods and used in most dietary supplements are the tocopherols. Tocopherols have

100

been recognized as potent antioxidants for many years. Since they stop the formation and progression of free radicals, researchers have speculated that they may also be useful in preventing or even treating cancer. Much research has been dedicated to this goal. While tocopherols are effective antioxidants and may help *prevent* the series of events that lead to the development of cancer, they have shown little promise in cancer treatment.[46] Once cancer has established a foothold, tocopherols have little effect. Only very large doses of tocopherols have shown to have anticancer effects, but at such large doses, healthy cells are adversely affected as well.

Tocotrienols from palm oil, however, have a far greater effect on cancer than their tocopherol cousins.[47] Unlike tocopherols, tocotrienols display potent anticancer activity at doses that have little or no effect on normal cell growth or function. At relatively small doses, tocotrienols can stop and even reverse the growth of tumors. Although tocotrienols have up to 60 times more antioxidant potency, most of their antitumor activity is independent of their antioxidant activity. The exact reason why tocotrienols are more potent than tocopherols is not completely understood, but at least part of the reason seems to be because of greater cellular accumulation. Tocotrienols accumulate in tissues while tocopherols tend to concentrate more in the blood.

A number of recent studies have shown that tocotrienols, but not tocopherols, can exert direct inhibitory effects on cell growth in human cancer cells.[48-50] The inhibitory effect is most pronounced with gamma- and delta-tocotrienol.

It is thought that tocotrienols exert their antitumor activity by modulating a number of intracellular signaling pathways involved in mitogenesis (cell division) and apoptosis (programmed cell death) as well as enhancing the efficiency of the immune system.

Tocotrienols have shown to be effective against biologically induced, chemically induced, and injected/transplanted cancers.[51]

An example of the biologically induced cancer is one caused by a virus. Epstein-Barr virus is known to cause cancer and is often associated with breast cancer. Tocotrienols have been shown to inhibit tumor promotion by the Epstein-Barr virus.[52]

Researchers often induce cancer in lab animals using potent carcinogenic chemicals. Let's look at one study were liver cancer was

101

chemically induced in lab animals. Fourteen rats were used in the study. They were separated into two equal groups, one of which received tocotrienol supplementation. After 9 months the livers of all the animals were removed and examined. Tumors were found in all 7 of the animals that did not receive tocotrienols whereas only 1 out of the 7 that did receive tocotrienols showed evidence of cancer.[53] This equated to an 86 percent success rate in preventing cancer.

In other studies human cancer cells are injected or implanted into lab animals. This way, researchers can see how experimental treatments actually affect the types of cancer found in humans. In all cases tocotrienols effectively knock out the cancerous cells.

A large number of studies have demonstrated the anticancer effects of palm oil tocotrienols, particularly in the treatment of breast cancer. Researchers Sumit Shah and Paul Sylvester of the College of Pharmacy at the University of Louisiana state: "These findings suggest that tocotrienols may have significant value as therapeutic agents for breast cancer prevention and/or treatment."[54] Palm oil tocotrienols not only help prevent cancer, but as these researchers have stated, may also be useful in cancer treatment.

Researchers have identified a number of nutrients in various fruits and vegetables that fight cancer. Some of these have great potential as therapeutic agents that can be used in cancer treatment. How do tocotrienols measure up? Cancer researcher Yoshihisa Yano and colleagues at Osaka City University Medical School, in Japan, state that "Tocotrienols are one of the most potent anticancer agents of all natural compounds."[55] Wow! That's a pretty strong statement. If true, since red palm oil has the highest naturally occurring concentration of tocotrienols, it would make it one of the best cancer fighting foods we could eat.

Other researchers agree. Palm oil added into the diet can have a significant protective effect. N. Guthrie and colleagues at in the departments of biochemistry and oncology at the University of Western Ontario state: "Experiments in our laboratory have shown that tocotrienols inhibit proliferation and growth of [cancer] cells....These results suggest that diets containing palm oil may reduce the risk of breast cancer." Guthrie recommends the use of palm oil and/or tocotrienols as a part of the protocol in treating breast cancer. His research has shown that combining palm oil tocotrienols with standard anticancer therapies such as Tamoxifen enhances the effectiveness of the treatment.[56]

Apoptosis

One way tocotrienols defeat cancer is by stimulating the body's own natural anticancer defense mechanisms. They do this is by inducing apoptosis or programmed death in the cancerous cells. Tocotrienols activate enzymes in cancerous cells that cause the cells to break apart or self destruct. This is a completely natural and harmless defense against cancer. Unlike radiation and chemotherapy, healthy cells remain unaffected.

Apoptosis is a normal and natural form of cell death or cell suicide in which a genetically programmed sequence of events leads to the elimination of cells. This process occurs without releasing any harmful substances into the surrounding area, so other cells are not adversely affected. Apoptosis plays a crucial role in developing and maintaining health by eliminating old, unnecessary, and unhealthy cells and replacing them with new ones. Apoptosis occurs in each one of us on a continual basis. The human body replaces perhaps a million cells a second.

When cells become cancerous, normal processes are disrupted. Normal signals to initiate programmed cell death do not occur. Consequently, cancer cells essentially become immortal. If given the opportunity, such as in a lab where they can be given a continual supply of nutrients, they would live and continue to grow indefinitely. Much of the cancer research that is currently being done uses cancer cells that were originally harvested from the host decades ago. Some cancer lines go back as far as the 1950s.

Apoptosis is initiated by special enzymes (caspases) that are present in all cells, including cancer cells. In cancer cells, however, genetic signaling has gone haywire and these enzymes are never activated. Tocotrienols kick start the signaling process that activates the enzymes that initiates apoptosis.

Apoptosis is an important aspect of normal mammary gland growth and remodeling as well as a mechanism for eliminating cancerous cells from the breast. Extensive research on human breast cancer cells has shown tocotrienols from palm oil (principally gamma- and delta-tocotrienols) initiate apoptosis in diseased cells.[57-63]

Ordinary vitamin E (i.e., alpha-tocopherol) does not induce programmed cell death in cancer cells.[64] Even very high doses of alpha-tocopherol have no effect on cancer cell apoptosis.[65]

Immune System

The immune system plays an essential role in maintaining overall health and in fighting cancer. When cancer develops, it's the white blood cells of the immune system that go into action to eliminate the threat. How fast and how far the cancer develops depends to a large extent on the efficiency of your immune system.

Palm oil enhances the immune system and aids in antibody production, thus taking an active role in supporting the immune system in fighting cancer.[66] The antitumor effect of palm oil is believed in part to be due to improved immune function. Both vitamin E and carotenes support the immune system in fighting cancer.[67-69]

Consumption of tocopherols and tocotrienols affect the proliferation of lymphocytes (white blood cells) located in the lymph nodes. Evidence suggests that white blood cells known as natural killer (NK) cells increase in lab animals supplemented with tocotrienols and implanted with human breast cancer cells. Some researchers believe tocotrienols mimic the effects of or induce the production of interferon, which stimulates immune blood cells to fight cancer.

Beta-carotene has been reported to have immune modulatory effects, in particular, enhancement of natural killer cell activity and tumor necrosis factor production by macrophages (another type of white blood cell). Studies show that palm oil carotene increases activity of white blood cells (natural killer cells and B-lymphocytes) and suppresses the growth of human cancer cells.[70]

REDUCING RISK OF CANCER WITH PALM OIL

Most of the studies mentioned in this chapter focus on specific components of red palm oil such as tocotrienols and carotenes. In some of these studies the amount of the substances used was much higher than that contained in a typical serving of palm oil. One might ask, in order to get the same amount of protection demonstrated in studies is it necessary to consume massive amounts of oil? The answer is "no." All of the anticancer and antioxidant substances within red palm oil work together synergistically to enhance the oil's effectiveness. So the consumption of a serving or two of red palm oil a day can be very beneficial.

Instead of adding more oil into your diet, it is better to replace some or all of the fat you ordinarily use with palm oil. This way your total fat intake won't change, but the benefit you receive can be significant.

The effect of replacing other oils with red palm oil on cancer incidence was clearly demonstrated in one notable study.[71] In this study 100 rats were separated into five groups of 20. The animals were put on a 20 percent fat diet with each group containing a different type of fat: corn oil, soybean oil, red palm oil, RBD (refined) palm oil, and metabisulfite-treated palm oil. As you recall from previous chapters, RBD palm oil is a refined, bleached, and deodorized oil. It's also known as white palm oil. Refining removes practically all the carotenes and some of the vitamin E. Metabisulfite is a common preservative added to foods to prevent oxidation. In palm oil it also helps to retain some of the carotenes during processing. Researchers wanted to see how a diet containing each of these oils affects tumor growth and development.

The food given to the animals was identical except for the type of fat. The food also contained 7, 12-dimethylbenz(a)anthracene (DMBA) a very potent carcinogenic chemical. It is a favorite for researchers wanting to chemically induce cancer in test animals because it is so powerful, tumors develop within just a few weeks. DMBA is far more toxic than any chemical normally encountered in our environment and, under ordinary circumstances, produces terminal cancer at a rate of 100 percent in a very short time. The animals remained on the diet for 5 months.

The animals all developed cancerous tumors at different rates according to the type of oil in their diet. At autopsy it was found that the rats which were fed corn and soybean oils had significantly more tumors than those on the three palm oil diets. This demonstrated that *all* the palm oils were protective. Even the refined white palm oil and the refined palm oil with metabisulfite protected the animals against cancer better than the two polyunsaturated oils.

Although corn and soybean oils contained a larger amount of tocopherols than palm oil, they contain virtually no tocotrienols. Red palm oil produced the lowest number of tumors. The corn oil group had nearly three times as many tumors as the red palm oil group. The soybean oil had over twice as many tumors.

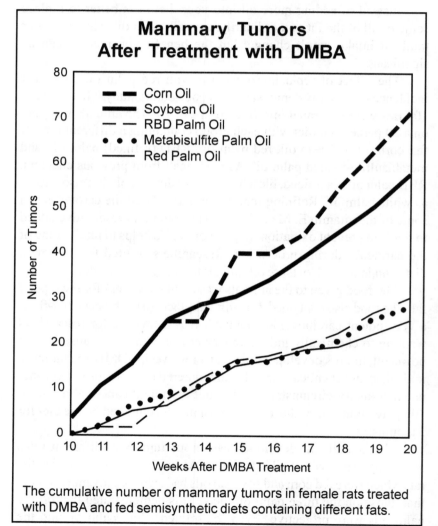

The cumulative number of mammary tumors in female rats treated with DMBA and fed semisynthetic diets containing different fats.

Total number of tumors in the corn oil group after 20 weeks was 71, soybean oil 57, RBD palm oil 30, metabisulfite treated palm oil 28, and red palm oil 25.

Several other studies have shown that when palm oil is added into the diet, it reduces the risk of cancer and prolongs lifespan.[72-74] It doesn't matter if the primary fat in the diet is soybean oil, corn oil, lard, or beef tallow, when palm oil is added or replaces these other oils, cancer incidence declines.

Palm oil contains a mixture of anticancer antioxidants. It is like an anti-cancer dietary supplement that you can take by the spoonful or use in everyday food preparation and cooking.

Daily use of palm oil can help prevent cancer. It can also be helpful in treating active cancer as well. The high nutrient content of red palm oil tempers the devastating side effects often accompanying conventional cancer treatment. People have reported that when they used red palm oil during cancer treatment, they do not experience excessive hair loss, nausea, bleeding gums, and other side effects commonly associated with chemotherapy and radiation. The antioxidant nutrients and radiation blocking effects of squalene in the oil protects against these harmful effects and assists in boosting the immune system in the fight to eradicate the cancer.

SKIN CANCER

The incidence of skin cancer has greatly increased over the past few decades. Currently about 3 million cases of skin cancer occur globally each year. One in every three cancers diagnosed is skin cancer. According to statistics from the American Cancer Society one in every five Americans will develop skin cancer in their lifetime.

The three most common forms of skin cancer are basal cell carcinoma, squamous cell carcinoma, and malignant melanoma. Of the three, malignant melanoma is by far the most dangerous. Although less prevalent than the other two, it is the major cause of death from skin cancer. One out of every four cases of melanoma becomes fatal. The increase in incidence of skin cancer and particularly melanoma is alarming. Since 1980 the incidence of melanoma has tripled.

Researchers have found that diet and lifestyle changes can prevent at least two-thirds of all skin cancers. While many factors may be involved, some researchers believe the increase in skin cancer is due primarily to the trend of replacing saturated fats in the diet with polyunsaturated fats. The fats that we eat are incorporated into skin tissues. Polyunsaturated fats are very unstable and easily oxidized by ultraviolet (UV) radiation from the sun and oxygen in the air. When polyunsaturated fats in the skin oxidize, they form free radicals that can damage the DNA in cells, causing cancer to form. Since the 1980s polyunsaturated fat consumption has nearly doubled, while saturated fat consumption has steadily declined.[75] The increase in polyunsaturated fat consumption parallels the increase in skin cancer.

Doctors believe that exposure to UV radiation is the most important factor in causing skin cancer. Overexposure to sunlight and repeated incidences of sunburn increase the risk of skin cancer. Polyunsaturated fats in the skin increase our sensitivity to the sun and make us more vulnerable to sunburn. This explains why skin cancer has been on the rise since the 1980s when the push by the vegetable oil industry succeeded in replacing tropical oils and other saturated fats with processed vegetable oils and hydrogenated fats.

It is interesting to note that in Malaysia and Indonesia which straddle the equator and where sun exposure is intense, skin cancer is relatively rare. Both countries also happen to produce and consume large amounts of palm oil. A large part of the population works outdoors exposed to the hot tropical sun every single day, yet sun exposure has not caused an epidemic of skin cancer like what is happening in other parts of the world. For example, Australia has a climate ranging from temperate to tropical. Although the climate on a whole is much less intense than Malaysia and Indonesia and more people work indoors protected from the sun, Australia has the highest skin cancer rates in the world. Australians eat essentially no palm oil, but consume primarily canola and soybean oils.

Our increasing dependence on junk foods and packaged convenience foods and our general avoidance of fresh fruits and vegetables has also contributed to the problem. Fruits and vegetables are the source of most of the antioxidant nutrients in our diet. Consequently, our antioxidant defenses are seriously weakened. Poor antioxidant status leaves us more vulnerable to free radicals and the destruction they cause.

Our diet has a direct impact on the health of our skin. Foods rich in antioxidants increase the antioxidant levels present in the skin. One of the most important antioxidants in our skin is vitamin E. On average the vitamin E in our skin is comprised of about 87 percent alpha-tocopherol, 9 percent gamma-tocopherol, 3 percent gamma-tocotrienol, and 1 percent alpha-tocotrienol. These values, of course, vary depending on each individual's diet. The scarcity of tocotrienols present in the skin reflects the minute amount of this vitamin in the average diet. Consuming foods rich in tocotrienols, such as palm oil, can increase the amount of this nutrient in our skin, thus providing us with a greater degree of protection from the processes that cause skin cancer.

After consumption, tocotrienols are absorbed from the intestinal tract into the bloodstream. However, they do not remain in the bloodstream for long. They quickly migrate into the tissues of the body and especially the skin, where they can accumulate in relatively large amounts.[76] Tocotrienol concentrations in the skin and fat tissues can be tenfold to that in the blood.[77, 78] Simply consuming palm oil can greatly increase the amount of protective tocotrienols in your skin.

Our bodies excrete oil through the sebaceous glands located near the hair follicles on our skin. This oil is called sebum. Sebum serves as a transport mechanism taking vitamin E from the blood to the skin surface. Sebum lubricates the skin, makes it soft and flexible, and establishes a protective environment that blocks harmful UV radiation and infections from microorganisms.

Sebum enriched with tocotrienols can provide a great deal of protection from cancer. Since free radicals are involved in every step of the process of cancer development, researchers are now recommending antioxidant strategies as a solution to the prevention and therapy of skin cancer.[79]

Vitamin E isn't the only antioxidant in palm oil that protects the skin from cancer. Beta-carotene applied topically on the skin has also been found to significantly inhibit the growth of cancerous tumors.[80] Some studies show that not only does beta-carotene stop cancer from growing, but it reduces the size of the tumors as well.[81]

Another anticancer nutrient in palm oil that you learned about in Chapter 4 is squalene. Like tocotrienols, squalene is a potent antioxidant that has an affinity for the skin. The body's sebum contains a significant amount of squalene, which can be enhanced by the regular consumption of red palm oil. The added benefit of squalene is its remarkable ability to block the harmful effects UV radiation.

Consuming palm oil isn't the only way to increase the amount of tocotrienols in the skin. You can also apply it directly on the skin. Use it like a massage oil or moisturizer and rub it into the skin. Studies show that applying palm oil topically can help protect the skin from damaging oxidation that accelerates aging and promotes cancer.[82]

UV radiation destroys antioxidants in the skin. However prior application of palm oil to the skin preserves antioxidant status, protects against lipid peroxidation skin damage, and reduces risk of skin cancer.[83]

Palm oil protects against the damaging effects of free radicals regardless of how they are caused. A potent cancer causing chemical, 12-0- tetradecanoyl-phorbol-13-acetate (TPA), is used by researchers to induce skin cancer in lab animals. TPA is a powerful oxidant that generates free radicals. However, palm oil counters the oxidizing effects of TPA, protecting the body's antioxidant defenses from depletion. Applying palm oil to the skin prior to application of TPA has shown to significantly reduce the number and severity of tumors caused by this chemical.[84]

Because of palm oil's ability to protect the skin, a palm oil product called Palm Tocotrienol Rich Fraction (Palm TRF) is now gaining popularity as an ingredient in cosmetic formulations. Some of the cosmetics you use may already contain it.

Chapter 7

A Health Tonic

Palm oil can affect your health in so many positive ways it can be regarded as a health tonic. The fatty acids, antioxidants, and phytonutrients combine to provide many health benefits. In this chapter you will learn how palm oil can affect the health of your entire body by improving blood circulation and the delivery of oxygen to vital tissues and organs. You will also see how palm oil can help with specific health issues such as diabetes and neurological (brain and nerve) problems and how it protects and supports the function of vital organs such as the liver and lungs.

LIFEBLOOD OF THE BODY
Blood Circulation

Blood has long been regarded as the seat of life and vitality. Indeed, without it you would be dead. With too little blood or if blood flow were impeded, you would be less than healthy. Any degree of restriction of proper blood flow can be harmful. Our blood is literally the life-giving force or lifeblood of our bodies. It supplies all the cells throughout our body with the nutrients they need to carry on life and protect us from disease. The health of the blood can affect the health of every cell and every organ in the body.

The main function of the blood is to act as the body's transport system. It delivers oxygen, nutrients, hormones, and enzymes throughout the body and removes waste and toxins. Nearly half of the volume of blood consists of cells, which include red blood cells (erythrocytes), white blood cells (leukocytes), and platelets (thrombocytes). The remainder is a fluid called plasma, which contains dissolved proteins, sugars, fats, vitamins, and minerals. Red blood cells are by far the most numerous and give blood its distinctive red color. The primary function of red blood cells is to carry oxygen from the lungs to the tissues, where it is exchanged for the waste product carbon dioxide. White blood cells are the workforce of our immune system and play an important part in the defense against infection. Platelets are essential to arrest bleeding and repair damaged blood vessels. When an injury occurs, platelets clump together to begin the process of blood clotting.

The heart pumps blood into the lungs, where red blood cells exchange carbon dioxide for oxygen. Oxygenated blood then flows throughout the body. The blood vessels carrying oxygenated blood are called arteries. As the arteries travel away from the heart, they branch out and become smaller and smaller until they become so small that they are about the size of the red blood cells. These microscopic blood vessels are called capillaries. Passage through the capillaries is so narrow that blood cells must pass though one at a time in single file. Oxygen is released from the red blood cells and carbon dioxide is picked up in the capillaries. As the red blood cells absorb carbon dioxide, they head back to the lungs, traveling in blood vessels called veins.

Oxygen is vital to life. If you were denied oxygen for just a few minutes, you would suffocate and die. Likewise, our cells need oxygen. Every cell in the body requires a continual supply of oxygen to live. Our blood carries life-giving oxygen to all the cells and organs. If blood flow is hindered, oxygen cannot effectively reach cells. These cells die. If enough cells in an organ die from oxygen starvation, the entire organ can die or become severely crippled. When blood going to the heart is blocked, the heart begins to die. A heart attack results. When blood going to the brain is blocked, this leads to a stroke. When blood going to the kidneys is blocked, kidney failure can result. When blood going to the retina of the eye is blocked, retinopathy results. When blood going to the feet and legs is blocked, severe leg ischemia (localized obstruction of blood) results, leading to gangrene.

Blood flow doesn't need to be completely blocked to cause damage. Restricting blood flow can reduce oxygen delivery to the point that cells are constantly starved for oxygen. Just as our health would begin to fail if we were placed in an environment lacking an adequate amount of oxygen, our cells and organs respond in a similar way. When blood flow to the brain is hampered it can lead to dementia and other neurological problems.

Blood Cell Rigidity

Every organ in the body contains an intricate system of capillaries to bring it life-giving oxygen and carry away waste. Because the capillaries are so narrow, blood cells must literally squeeze through them. This requires that blood cells be flexible enough to pass easily through the capillaries. A condition that is associated with many health problems is the loss of elasticity or deformability in blood cells which prevents them from traveling easily though capillaries. Blood cells that become too rigid may clog narrow passageways, preventing the delivery of oxygen as well as glucose and other nutrients to the cells and organs. Carbon dioxide and toxins are not adequately removed, which can poison surrounding cells. The loss of blood cell elasticity can create an environment ideal for disease.

White blood cells are our immune cells. They fight off infections and dispose of toxins. These cells are very flexible, which allows them to squeeze though tiny spaces and cross through capillary walls. Their membranes are fluid enough that they can completely surround a germ and engulf it. If the membrane of the white blood cell becomes too stiff, it can not function properly. Your immune system would suffer.

Red blood cells need to be flexible enough to pass easily through the capillaries and deliver their load of oxygen. Since 40 percent of the volume of blood is composed of red blood cells, the action of these cells plays an important role in our health. If they become too rigid, they can pool in parts of the body. These areas become oxygen starved which can result in tissue death or disease.

One of the first symptoms associated with the loss of blood cell deformability is elevated blood pressure. As blood cells become trapped, blood flow is impeded. Blood pressure builds. Increased blood pressure, in turn, increases the risk of heart disease, stroke, kidney disease, and puts a strain on the entire body.

Cells deprived of oxygen and other nutrients become sick and die. The organs and tissues that are affected slowly degenerate or become diseased. Since each organ in the body is laced with a fine network of capillaries, a reduction in blood flow can affect any part of the body.

What Causes Blood Cell Rigidity?

Although many conditions contribute to the loss of blood cell flexibility, the primary cause is oxidative stress.[1] Polyunsaturated fatty acids and proteins within the cell membrane become oxidized. In this process the structure of these molecules is changed. Polyunsaturated fatty acids (PUFA) normally make cells more fluid. Saturated fatty acids and cholesterol give cells strength and elasticity. However, when polyunsaturated fatty acids become oxidized, they become rigid. This causes the cell to stiffen and lose its ability to deform and move freely through capillaries.

Saturated fats, being resistant to oxidation, do not harden. In fact, they can act as antioxidants and prevent oxidation. When polyunsaturated fatty acids are surrounded by saturated fatty acids, they are protected to some degree from oxidation. Therefore, cells that are composed primarily of saturated fat and cholesterol protect PUFA from oxidation. However, when cells absorb too many PUFA from a diet high in polyunsaturated vegetable oils, the cells can become vulnerable.

Normally the body's antioxidant enzymes protect PUFAs from oxidation. But if the diet is low in antioxidant nutrients, this protection is lacking. Many people's diets are sadly deficient in antioxidants. Most of the foods we eat are highly processed and nutrient deficient. The primary food in our diet is white flour and white rice, both of which have been stripped of most of their nutrients. Sugar consumption has risen from about 5 pounds a year a century ago to around 150 pounds today. Sugar supplies no vitamins or minerals but drains them from the body as they are metabolized. Polyunsaturated oils also burn up antioxidants, thus lowering our antioxidant status.

Too many polyunsaturated fatty acids or too little saturated fat and cholesterol in blood cell membranes make them weak and fragile.

Factors that Affect Blood Cell Flexibility

Studies show that flexibility and strength of red and white blood cells are reduced by many factors, some of which are:

- Low antioxidant status. Diet lacking adequate fruits and vegetables.[3-6]
- Diet high in polyunsaturated oils.[7, 8]
- Diet high in canola oil.[9]
- Elevated blood glucose levels (i.e., diet high in simple carbohydrates).[10, 11]
- Excessive prooxidants in the diet or environment (i.e. smog, cigarette smoke, food additives, etc.).[12, 13]
- Low immunity and frequent infections.[14, 15]
- Drugs (e.g. aspirin, morphine, antidiabetic drugs, cholesterol-lowering drugs).[16-18]
- Alcohol.[19]
- Stress or trauma.[20, 21]
- Age.[22]

Saturated fat and cholesterol keep the membranes strong and elastic. Reducing the normal amount of cholesterol in cell membranes can be fatal, not only to the cell but to us as well. Studies which inhibit the absorption of cholesterol into cell membranes show that the cell's function and lifespan are seriously reduced. Canola oil is exceptionally harmful to blood cell stability. Canola oil is known to block cholesterol uptake into cell membranes. This characteristic alters strength and elastic properties of blood cells, significantly shortening the lifespan of animals fed canola oil.[2]

Palm Oil Preserves Blood Cell Flexibility

Reducing the amount of polyunsaturated fats in the diet and replacing them with palm oil can help protect you from many of the health problems created by stiffened blood cells. The saturated fat in palm oil protects polyunsaturated fatty acids in blood cells from oxidation and provides the cell membranes with strength and elasticity.

The antioxidants in red palm oil help protect vulnerable polyunsaturated fatty acids in cell membranes from oxidation and preserve cell deformability.[23]

Saturated fats, including palm oil, have been criticized as contributing to heart disease by clogging the arteries. Yet ironically, palm oil does just the opposite, it *improves* blood circulation by protecting cell membranes and preserving blood cell flexibility.

Blood cell elasticity plays an important role in heart health. Blood cell rigidity increases blood pressure which is a major risk factor for heart disease. Research indicates that loss of blood cell deformability may be a precursor to heart attack and stroke.[24]

Reduced blood flow to the brain can contribute to mental and emotional degeneration. Researchers have found correlations between blood cell rigidity and senile dementia, Alzheimer's disease, and schizophrenia.[25, 26]

Reduced blood cell deformability is associated with a variety of other conditions including obesity, asthma, bacterial infections, alcoholism, severe trauma, diabetes, kidney disease, liver disease, and cancer.

NEUROLOGICAL DISORDERS

Modern medical technology has now made it possible to replace parts of the human body that are damaged or dysfunctional. Prosthetic legs and arms can restore movement and function. Artificial hips, kidney dialysis machines, and pacemakers aid weakened organs. Transplants can replace vital organs and tissues. There are replacements for just about every part of the body you can imagine with one major exception— the brain and spinal cord. You can live with a replacement leg, kidney, or heart, but you can't replace the brain. What you have must last your entire lifetime. Keeping our brains and our minds active and healthy is of great concern.

One of the things that affect neurological (nerve and brain) function is blood flow. Our brains require a constant supply of oxygen and glucose in order to function properly. Therefore, it is essential to have good circulation to the brain.

Palm oil can be regarded as "brain food" because it can help maintain proper blood flow, allowing the brain to receive the nutrients it needs. Arteries narrowed by swelling or plaque buildup hinder blood flow to the brain. Palm oil has been shown to increase blood circulation in arteries that feed the brain, thus helping to maintain brain health and prevent strokes.[27, 28] In this way palm oil can help keep our minds healthy by improving or maintaining proper blood flow.

Palm oil helps protect the brain another way. The brain is composed of about 60 percent fat and cholesterol. An adequate amount of fat in the diet helps to keep our minds sharp and memory clear and helps to keep us sane and mentally balanced. Too little fat in the diet can lead to depression, suicide, schizophrenia, and other neurological disorders. Low-fat dieting can promote neurological disturbances. A certain amount of fat is necessary in the diet for optimal mental function. Saturated fat is important because a large portion of the fat in our brains is and must be saturated. Palm oil provides a good source of fat for this purpose.

Because of the high percentage of lipids (fat and cholesterol) in nerve tissue, the brain is very susceptible to lipid peroxidation and free-radical induced degeneration. Saturated fat is needed for stability. The high saturated and monounsaturated fat content of palm oil along with its abundance of antioxidants helps protect the brain from lipid peroxidation.

Vitamin E, principally alpha-tocopherol, has shown to be effective in blocking the destructive action of free radicals. While any good source of vitamin E may help protect the brain from oxidative damage, palm oil is of particular interest. Studies have shown that palm tocotrienols are significantly more effective than tocopherols in protecting the brain against damage caused by an assortment of oxidative toxins.[29] Tocotrienols not only protect fats in brain cells but also proteins.

Free radicals represent a major contributor to brain damage in disorders such as epilepsy[30] head trauma,[31] and ischemia stroke.[32, 33] Oxidative damage is also implicated in neurodegenerative diseases such as Huntington's, Alzheimer's, and Parkinson's disease.[34, 35]

Diet plays an important role in many neurological disorders. The foods we eat may either protect or harm the brain. The dramatic increase in Alzheimer's, Parkinson's, and other neurological disorders over the past few decades appears to be related to the increasing amount of processed and devitalized foods in our diet.

Our foods nowadays are loaded with neurotoxins—substances that damage nerve and brain cells. One of these is glutamate. Glutamate is an amino acid that can cause nerve and brain damage. It is one of several neurotoxins commonly used as a food additive. The primary sources of glutamate come from monosodium glutamate (MSG), aspartame (Nutrasweet), hydrolyzed vegetable protein, and soy protein extract. If you look at the ingredients label of food in the store, you may be surprised to find these additives in a huge number of foods, particularly packaged and convenience foods. Even so-called "health foods" often contain these substances so getting too much is not only a possibility, but for many people it is a reality.

Glutamate-containing substances are added to foods to stimulate our senses and enhance flavor. Eating too much glutamate can over-stimulate or excite nerve cells to such a degree that they become exhausted and die. For this reason, glutamate is known as an excitotoxin. Numerous studies have shown that glutamate interferes with brain function and kills brain cells.[36] Studies have also shown that glutamate-induced cell death increases the level of destructive free radicals in the brain, thus causing further harm. High levels of glutamate have been found associated with various neurological conditions including Alzheimer's disease, Huntington's disease, and Lou Gehrig's disease.

Glutamate toxicity is intensified by the accompanying production of free radicals. Antioxidants then can help quench the destructive action of glutamate. Researchers studying the effect that glutamate has in causing brain cell death have found that tocotrienols in palm oil prevent glutamate-induced cell death. Palm oil eaten even as long as six hours after consuming glutamate will stop the destructive action of this neurotoxin.[37]

Besides oxidative damage, glutamate interferes with cell communication, activating processes within cells that leads to their death. Studies show that tocotrienols, in addition to their antioxidant properties, also protect brain cells from glutamate-induced death by regulating cell communication.

Foods rich in vitamin E may not be of much help. Studies show that alpha-tocopherol, the type most commonly found in our diet does not block glutamate-induced death. However, alpha-tocotrienol in palm oil does. In laboratory studies tocotrienol-treated neurons maintain healthy growth and motility even in the presence of excess glutamate. Researchers have found that alpha-tocotrienol protects the brain from other neurotoxins such as homocysteine and 1-buthionine sulfoximine.[38]

Glutamate in one form or another is found in a wide variety of foods, especially in restaurants, so it is almost impossible to avoid. Using palm oil on a regular basis can help block the destructive action of glutamate and other neurotoxins in our foods.

Tocotrienols may have a normalizing effect on the brain and nervous system. Some doctors are prescribing tocotrienol supplements in the treatment of neurological disorders. For instance one lady reports remarkable improvement in her son. "My 20-year-old son has intractable epilepsy. He did not develop seizures until the age of eight. At eleven they became uncontrollable and he suffered significant brain injury. He is now about 80 percent controlled with a regime of anticonvulsant medications and vitamins, including a tocotrienol complex from palm oil. The neurologist and I knew we are on to something with this supplement. His improvement has been remarkable. My son is even regaining cognitive skills!"

The mind is a terrible thing to lose. Adding palm oil into your diet is a simple measure you can take to help protect your brain from harm and keep it healthy.

DIABETES

Our cells are like little engines. They run on fuel and perform tasks. Their duties vary, depending on the types of cells they are. Muscle cells give us the ability to move, nerve cells carry messages, liver cells produce bile, pancreatic cells produce insulin, and so forth. In order for an engine to function, it needs an adequate supply of fuel. The same is true for our cells. The fuel our cells use is sugar, more specifically, glucose. Glucose is also called "blood sugar." Our cells need a continual supply of glucose to keep them alive and functioning.

Glucose is carried in the bloodstream to all the cells in the body. If cells are unable to get the glucose they need, they literally starve to death. If we don't get enough to eat we become weak, sick, and could die. Our cells are the same way. If they don't get enough glucose, they become weak, sick, and die. If enough cells in any particular organ become sick and dysfunctional then the entire organ becomes sick and dysfunctional, consequently the whole body is affected.

Cells can be deprived of glucose in several ways. One way is to restrict or cut off blood flow to a certain area of the body. Cells in that area are deprived of both glucose as well as oxygen. An example of this is in an artery plugged with plaque.

Another way is if a person is in a severe state of starvation. Obviously, if a person isn't consuming food, the cells aren't getting nourishment either. Skipping a meal or two or getting little food for an extended amount of time occurs frequently. The body has mechanisms in place that protect us in such circumstances. If we don't eat enough food to supply the glucose our cells need, fatty acids stored in our fat cells can be used as an alternative fuel to glucose.

A third and very important situation which deprives cells of energy is when the cells have difficulty absorbing glucose from the bloodstream. This is the situation in type 2 diabetes.

Cells cannot absorb glucose or fatty acids directly from the bloodstream. They need a helper. This helper is insulin. Insulin is a hormone that unlocks the door in the cell membrane that allows glucose and fatty acids to enter. The pancreas manufactures insulin and regulates the amount of insulin in the blood. When we eat a meal, much of the food is broken down and converted into glucose and released into the bloodstream. After a meal, blood sugar rises sharply. In response, the pancreas pumps out insulin. Insulin pulls the glucose out of the blood and puts it into the cells, where it is used to produce energy. As blood sugar drops, insulin levels fall back to normal levels.

The two most common types of diabetes are type 1 and type 2. Type 1 occurs when the pancreas is unable to produce enough insulin to meet the body's needs. In type 2 diabetes the pancreas may be able to produce a normal amount of insulin, but the body's cells have become unresponsive to it. This is referred to as insulin resistance.

In type 2 diabetes a higher amount of insulin is needed to pass glucose from the bloodstream into the cells. In this situation blood sugar levels can rise very high and remain elevated for an extended amount of time. As blood sugar levels return to normal, insulin levels drop and delivery of glucose into the cells slows down. Because the cells are resistant to insulin, glucose delivery is greatly hampered, especially between meals when insulin levels are lowest. Many cells are starving for energy. Cells unable to get the energy they need sicken and die. Sick and dying cells in artery walls and in capillaries promote inflammation, blood clotting, and plaque formation.

Diabetics also have a problem with "hard" blood. Blood cells that become too stiff or rigid clog the circulatory system.[39] Red and white blood cells in diabetics have a decreased ability to bend and fit through small capillary passageways. They have a tendency to block the capillaries, cutting off circulation and raising blood pressure. As blood cells become more rigid, the microcirculation in organs and peripheral tissues is hindered.

Lipid peroxidation of polyunsaturated fatty acids in blood cell membranes causes loss of cell deformability and fluidity, leading to capillary blockage and reduction in blood circulation. This is a major factor leading to the complications seen in both type 1 and type 2 diabetes.[40, 41] These complications include high blood pressure, nerve damage (neuropathy), blindness (retinopathy), gangrene and amputation (peripheral vascular disease), and kidney failure (nephronpathy).

Reducing lipid peroxidation can help protect diabetics from these complications.[42-47] Replacing polyunsaturated vegetable fat with healthy saturated fats, such as palm oil, is one step you can take. Eating a diet rich in antioxidant nutrients and even taking antioxidant supplements can also protect against oxidation and free radical damage that cause loss of cell deformability.[48, 49]

Alpha-tocotrienol in palm oil is a powerful antioxidant that has been shown to protect blood cells from oxidative damage that causes loss of elasticity.[50] Therefore, replacing polyunsaturated vegetable oils with red palm oil can help protect your blood cells from oxidation and maintain proper circulation throughout the body.

One of the defining characteristics of type 2 diabetes is insulin resistance. Both animal and human studies show that diets high in trans fats, polyunsaturated fats, and refined carbohydrates promote insulin resistance. The effect is greatest when the diet is high in all three. In fact, when researchers want to induce diabetes in lab animals, they can do so by either feeding them a high carbohydrate diet[51, 52] or a high polyunsaturated fat diet.[53]

121

All of the major health problems associated with diabetes can be reduced by adding palm oil into the diet. The primary saturated fatty acids found in palm oil—palmitic, myristic, and stearic acids—have been shown to stimulate the transport of glucose from the bloodstream into the cells and, therefore, reverse insulin resistance.[54] Saturated fat, particularly from palm oil, increases delivery of glucose into cells. Monounsaturated and polyunsaturated fats do not.

Ironically, some people have criticized saturated fats as causing or at least contributing to insulin resistance. In their zeal to put blame on saturated fats, they point to studies showing insulin sensitivity decreasing in animals fed large amounts of saturated fat. What they conveniently fail to mention is that once a normal diet is resumed, insulin sensitivity returns to normal. It is a temporary effect and actually a self-governing safety mechanism.

Saturated fat stimulates glucose transport into cells; as the cells fill with glucose, a signal is sent to slow down entry of additional glucose. Excess glucose can be as harmful as too little. When the cells approach glucose saturation, a safety mechanism kicks in that slows down entry of glucose into the cells. In a sense, this could be called a state of *temporary* insulin resistance. What these studies show is that saturated fatty acids improve glucose transport as they are added into the diet, but on prolonged exposure they induce insulin resistance as a self regulatory mechanism to prevent harm from excessive glucose absorption. This type of insulin restriction is not harmful, but protective because it properly regulates how much glucose enters the cell.

PUFAs on the other hand do not improve insulin transport but block it, creating a different type of insulin resistance, the type that is harmful because it prevents the cells from getting adequate nourishment. This is the type of insulin resistance that is seen in diabetics.

You can induce diabetes in animals and humans by feeding them a diet high in polyunsaturated vegetable oils or sugar or both. But you cannot induce diabetes with a high saturated fat diet. It just won't happen. The type of insulin restriction resulting from a high polyunsaturated fat diet and high saturated fat diet is as different as night and day.

It is interesting that the Indians who lived on the Great Plains in the central part of the United States lived for generations on a diet dominated by meat and saturated fat. On this high saturated fat diet they never experienced diabetes. After living on reservations where they were given foods consisting of sugar, white flour, and processed vegetable oils, diabetes has become a serious problem. The same thing happened to the Eskimo. When they lived off the land, their diet consisted of 80 percent fat, mostly saturated. After living on permanent settlements where they were introduced to processed vegetable oils, white flour, and sweets, diabetes surfaced for the first time in their population. Again we see this happen among Pacific islanders. In some of these island populations the natural diets consist of up to 50 percent saturated fat, primarily from coconut. When these islanders move to New Zealand and other urbanized areas and reduce their saturated fat intake and start consuming processed vegetable oils and other modernized foods, many of them encounter diabetes for the first time.

Obesity is associated with an increased risk of diabetes. People who are overweight have a higher chance of becoming diabetic than those of normal weight. Eighty percent of diabetics are overweight. Overweight people tend to eat the wrong types of foods high in sugar, refined carbohydrates, vegetable oils, margarines, and low in fresh fruits and vegetables. Some people don't eat any vegetables at all except fried potatoes, which are often cooked in hydrogenated vegetable oil. With a diet like this, antioxidant status is severely compromised and polyunsaturated fat intake high. So oxidation of PUFA in cell membranes is bound to happen. Consequently, cells are going to become stiff. Both diabetes and obesity are associated with the loss of red blood cell flexibility.[55]

A low-fat diet is generally recommended for diabetes because fats are believed to increase the risk of obesity and heart disease. Limiting most fats, particularly vegetable oils and hydrogenated fats, is definitely a good thing. However, palm oil appears to be one of the best foods for diabetics.

Palm oil can help regulate blood sugar. Fats slow down digestion so that sugars are released into the bloodstream at a slower rate. This reduces the dramatic spike in blood sugar which is a major problem with diabetes.

Diabetics are counseled to eat foods with a low glycemic index. The glycemic index is an indicator of how much a food raises blood sugar levels. A food with a high glycemic index raises blood sugar levels more than one with a lower value. Sweet and starchy foods like white bread and sugar have high glycemic values. An index with a range of values between 0 to 100, pure glucose (sugar) has a glycemic value of 100—the maximum. Donuts come in at 76, apples 38, kidney beans (plain) 28. Palm oil has a glycemic index of 0. It does not raise blood sugar at all. When palm oil is added to other foods, it lowers the glycemic index of these foods, making them safer for diabetics to eat.

As you can see, palm oil can help improve blood circulation, protect against harmful free radicals, and normalize blood sugar and insulin levels. Anyone concerned about diabetes or blood sugar control should consider using palm oil as a part of their everyday diet.

LIVER DISEASE

The liver is one of the most important organs in the body. It performs literally hundreds of vital functions. It regulates, assembles, disassembles, and stores fats, proteins, and glucose. It absorbs oxygen and nutrients from the blood and balances the blood's glucose and amino-acid levels. It helps break down drugs and various toxins, and manufactures proteins, including blood proteins such as albumin and blood coagulation factors. The liver also produces bile, which removes waste products and helps digest fats in the small intestine.

Along with the kidneys, the liver acts to clear the blood of drugs and poisonous substances that would otherwise accumulate in the bloodstream. The liver absorbs the substances to be removed from the blood, alters their chemical structure, makes them water soluble, and excretes them in the bile.

The liver is involved in so many functions important to good health that, to put it simply: if your liver ain't happy, you ain't happy.

Because the liver is involved in so many vital functions, when it's diseased it can be life-threatening. Liver disease is a general term which can refer any liver disorder.

Hepatitis means inflammation of the liver; it may be caused by viruses, bacteria, parasites, alcohol, toxins, cancer, or other factors. Poor dietary choices and excessive alcohol consumption can cause deposition of excess fat in the liver which clogs bile ducts and interferes with normal liver function. Fatty liver (steatosis) can lead to hepatitis. Hepatitis can progress to liver cirrhosis, a degenerative condition characterized by massive tissue destruction and scarring.

Liver failure is the complete loss of liver function. When hepatitis severely impairs liver function to the point that it affects other organs, such as the brain, it can lead to liver failure. It may also occur as the end result of advanced cirrhosis.

In many parts of the world the primary cause of liver disease is infections. In parts of Africa and Asia up to 20 percent of the population carries the hepatitis B virus. Aflatoxin, a poison produced by a fungus (*Aspergillus flavus*), often contaminates stored foods especially grains, peanuts, and cassava. Aflatoxin is believed to be one of the major factors responsible for the high incidence of liver disease in tropical Africa and Southeast Asia.

The most common cause of liver disease in the US and most other developed countries is excessive alcohol consumption. Alcohol related disorders, which include alcoholic hepatitis and cirrhosis, outnumber all other types of liver disorders by at least five to one. Alcohol, like any other toxin, is processed in the liver. Excessive alcohol consumption slowly poisons the liver.

Currently no drugs or treatments are effective in restoring health to a diseased liver. In the case of liver cancer, the patient can undergo surgery and take anticancer drugs to increase chances of survival. But there is no cure. And there is no cure for hepatitis or cirrhosis. If the cause of these conditions is from alcohol consumption, the only known treatment is abstinence. Allowing the body to heal itself is the only method doctors have. Feeding the patient a healthy diet that promotes good health is the best medicine. Fortunately, the liver has an amazing capacity to heal itself—if given the chance. Foods that promote good liver function can assist in this process. The best insurance against liver failure is prevention. Eating a diet that promotes good liver health will help protect it against disease.

The question now is: what foods support good liver health? Obviously those foods that promote good overall health, such as fresh fruits, vegetables, and whole grains and such, will also support the liver. But what about fats? The types of fats in your diet also play a significant role. Too much of the wrong types of fats can lead to liver disease.

Researchers have investigated the role of dietary fat on liver health. Their results were a surprise. When researchers began investigating the effect dietary fats on liver health, they were influenced by the anti-saturated fat sentiment prevalent among promoters of the lipid theory of heart disease. Researchers reasoned that if saturated fat was bad for the arteries and heart, it must be bad for the liver as well. They expected saturated fats to promote liver disease and polyunsaturated fats to protect against it. What they found was the complete opposite. Saturated fat protected against liver disease while polyunsaturated fats promoted it! Since this discovery many researchers have tested and retested this finding with the same results. It is now universally accepted that dietary saturated fats protect the liver from disease.

Let's look at some of these studies. Since alcohol is a potent toxin, liver studies often focus on the effects associated with alcohol induced liver disease. Feeding lab animals large amounts of alcohol is an easy way to cause hepatitis and cirrhosis. Studies published in the 1980s and early 1990s discovered that saturated fats, usually palm or coconut oils, protected the liver from alcohol induced injury. In 1994 researchers A. Nanji and colleagues proposed a new treatment for alcoholic liver disease.[56] This treatment was to enrich the diet in saturated fat! In their study they showed that palm oil could effectively decrease alcoholic liver injury. Palm oil not only prevents liver disease but is effective in reversing it as well. Since there is no other effective treatment for liver disease, this dietary approach offers a simple, inexpensive solution.

The saturated fat and antioxidant content of palm oil makes it especially effective in protecting the liver from alcohol-induced damage. One of major reasons why alcohol (and other toxins and microbial agents) damage the liver is that they produce destructive free radicals. Saturated fatty acids are resistant to lipid peroxidation and protect the liver. In contrast, polyunsaturated fats promote liver injury that leads to hepatitis and cirrhosis.

Numerous studies have compared the effects of saturated and polyunsaturated vegetable oils in association with alcohol induced liver disease. The results were the same. Saturated fats protect against injury and polyunsaturated oils promote it.[57]

In one study for instance, researchers induced alcoholic injury in lab animals. Those given vegetable oil (corn oil) all showed significant liver damage. Even those given fish oil all showed significant liver damage. Those given saturated fat showed no liver damage at all. The liver was completely protected from the harmful effects of the alcohol.[58]

Studies on red blood cell deformability and composition have also been investigated to evaluate the possible role they may play in liver disease. Researchers have found that in hepatitis and cirrhosis patients, red blood cells are significantly more rigid.[59] Consequently, they are too stiff to flow freely through the small capillaries of the liver, reducing the delivery of oxygen and nutrients to the organ and exasperating the problem. Replacing polyunsaturated fats in the diet with saturated fats improves circulation, promotes healing, and reverses liver damage.

Studies show that in addition to blocking the destructive action of free radicals, saturated fats, and palm oil in particular, encourage the release of hormones that aid in protecting the liver from alcoholic induced injury.[60]

Fatty liver, another problem of concern, can be caused by either excessive alcohol or food consumption. Obesity is also recognized as a cause for fatty liver. Fatty buildup on the liver, which contributes to liver injury, is also lessened with saturated fat. Studies show that dietary saturated fat reduces fat buildup in the liver, strengthens liver cells' resistance to oxidation, and reduces injury.[61]

Palm oil not only helps prevent damage but also aids in the healing process as well, even when the diet still contains harmful substances. For example, a diet enriched with palm oil has shown to reverse alcoholic liver injury despite continued administration of alcohol.[62] Palm oil effectively reverses alcohol-induced injury, inflammation, and fibrosis.

Because palm oil protects the liver from injury and aids in its repair, researchers are now recommending it as the treatment of choice for various types of liver disease.[63, 64]

The liver appears to have an affinity for saturated fat. Researchers have found that animal species with long life spans, such as humans, have a higher percentage of saturated fat in liver tissue. It is believed that the saturated fat content protects the liver from lipid peroxidation that can cause liver dysfunction. The body apparently selectively chooses saturated fats to be incorporated into liver tissue as a means of protecting the organ against oxidative damage and maintaining an appropriate environment for membrane functions.[65]

In summary, dietary palm oil is a good choice to support liver function and help protect it from disease.

RESPIRATORY HEALTH

The respiratory system includes the lungs and air passageways. The need for a constant supply of oxygen cannot be overstressed. Think of the panic you would experience if suddenly you could not breathe or the difficulty you would have performing daily tasks if you were always short of breath. A healthy respiratory system is vital to overall health.

The health of your lungs and bronchial tubes (air passageways) can be affected by your diet and the environment.

Our lungs are filled with millions of tiny air sacs called alveoli. It is in the alveoli that oxygen is exchanged for carbon dioxide. When we take a breath, air flows into the alveoli and our lungs expand. Alveoli are inflated like little balloons. Oxygen diffuses into the bloodstream and is replaced by carbon dioxide. As we exhale, the alveoli are compressed, forcing the air back out of the lungs expelling carbon dioxide.

The surface inside each of the alveoli is covered by a membrane called the surfactant. The purpose of the surfactant is to reduce surface tension and prevent the alveoli from collapsing. If the alveoli collapse, air cannot fill the cavity and the oxygen-carbon dioxide exchange cannot happen. Saturated fat is essential for the exchange of oxygen and carbon dioxide.

The primary component of the surfactant is a phospholipid called dipalmitoyl phosphatidylcholine. Phospholipids are composed of two fatty acids and a phosphate group. The fatty acids in this important phospholipid are both saturated, each of which are a palmitic acid, the type abundant in palm oil.

A deficiency or dysfunction of the surfactant can play a role in some respiratory diseases including chronic obstructive pulmonary disease, asthma, cystic fibrosis, interstitial lung disease, pneumonia, and alveolar proteinosis.

The inability to fully inflate the alveoli of the lungs results in respiratory distress. This condition is usually caused by impairment of

128

the surfactant in the alveoli. Infant respiratory distress syndrome (IRDS) is the most common form of this condition. The surfactant in newborns is not completely developed. IRDS often affects premature infants and can be life-threatening. In the United States, IRDS is the leading cause of death in premature infants, affecting 50,000 infants and resulting in over 5000 deaths each year.

Over the past three decades there has been an increase in the prevalence of asthma and allergic rhinitis in developed countries. This increase has occurred despite improved methods of treatment. Researchers believe that eating habits may be a key factor in the growing number of people affected by these conditions.

With the emphasis on reducing the intake of saturated fats and cholesterol, we eat more polyunsaturated fats. As a result, the amount of polyunsaturated linoleic acid incorporated into our bodies has increased from 8 to 15 percent. The increase in asthma and allergic rhinitis is paralleled by a fall in the consumption of saturated fat and an increase in polyunsaturated fat. Researchers postulate that displacing saturated fat with polyunsaturated fat in the diet is the primary factor in the rise of these conditions.[66, 67]

Increasing consumption of polyunsaturated vegetable oil has increased the amount of linoleic acid in the diet, which is converted into prostaglandins that increase allergic sensitization. In contrast, saturated fats do not promote inflammation or allergic sensitization.

The increased consumption of polyunsaturated fats affect the respiratory system in another way. Studies indicate that rigid red blood cells become trapped more easily in certain organs. The lungs, spleen, and liver are major organs where these cells are trapped and blood is pooled and blood flow decreased.[68] Patients with bronchial asthma show appreciable increase in red blood cell rigidity causing blockages in microvessels and preventing oxygen delivery and release of carbon dioxide.[69]

Another condition linked to the increasing use of polyunsaturated fats is lung cancer. The increase in the incidence of lung cancer is an interesting phenomenon. The number of Americans who smoke has been declining for the past 20 years. According to federal studies 20.9 percent of adults currently smoke. This is the lowest level since the early 1930s. Despite the decline in smoking, lung cancer continues to increase. The evidence linking tobacco smoke to lung cancer is indisputable so why has lung cancer rates continued to increase? One answer is that we have become more vulnerable to tobacco smoke because of a diet high in polyunsaturated fats and low in antioxidants.

Accumulating evidence suggests that dietary antioxidant vitamins are positively associated with lung function or lung health. Lung function can be evaluated by measuring what is called "vital capacity." The largest volume of air that can be moved in and out of the lungs is the vital capacity. The vital capacity measurement gives an indication of lung health. Studies show that vital capacity is greater with those who consume a higher percentage of antioxidants.[70]

Using palm oil in the diet in place of other vegetable oils can help strengthen your lungs and prevent respiratory problems.

DIGESTION AND NUTRIENT ABSORPTION

Fats aid in digestion and nutrient absorption. Fat slows down the passage of food from the stomach into the intestinal tract. There are several benefits to this. One benefit is that foods remain in contact with stomach acids and digestive enzymes for a longer amount of time, thus reducing the likelihood that harmful bacteria, viruses, and fungi will survive and be passed on to where they can do harm.

A second benefit of holding food in the stomach longer is that we feel satisfied for a longer amount of time before we feel hungry again. In this way we are less inclined to snack between meals and we feel less hungry at the next meal, thus reducing the consumption of excess calories we might otherwise consume. This principal is used in some of the popular low carb and moderately high fat diets that have become popular in recent years.[71]

Another benefit is that sugars are released into the bloodstream at a slower rate so there is less of an impact on blood sugar and insulin levels, an extremely important consideration for diabetics and others with blood sugar concerns.

Perhaps the most significant benefit of having food remain in the stomach longer is that it allows digestive enzymes and acids a longer amount of time to break down and release nutrients. Eating fat with meals actually increases the amount of nutrients you get out of your food. The effect of incorporating a sufficient amount of fat into the diet can have a very significant effect on nutrient availability and absorption and, consequently, your health.

Fat improves the availability and absorption of most all vitamins and minerals and is essential in order to properly absorb fat-soluble nutrients. The fat soluble vitamins include vitamins A, D, E, and K. Other fat soluble nutrients include alpha-carotene, beta-carotene and other carotenoids. These nutrients are absolutely vital to good health.

You can eat fruits and vegetables loaded with nutrients, but if you don't include fat you will only absorb a portion of them. Taking vitamin tablets won't help much because they too need fat to facilitate proper absorption. Eating a low-fat diet, therefore, can actually be detrimental.

How much of an affect does fat have on nutrient absorption? Apparently a lot. In a study conducted at Ohio State University, researchers looked at absorption of three carotenoids (beta-carotene, lycopene, and lutein) in meals that had added fat. The researchers used avocado, which is relatively high in monounsaturated fat, as their source of fat.

Eleven test subjects were given a meal of fat-free salsa and bread. On another day the same meal was given, but this time avocado was added to the salsa, boosting the fat content of the meal to about 37 percent of calories. Blood levels of the test subjects showed that beta-carotene increased by 2.6 times and lycopene 4.4 times. This indicated that adding a little fat to the meal can more than double, triple, or quadruple nutrient absorption.

A second test involved eating a salad. The first salad included romaine lettuce, baby spinach, shredded carrots, and a non-fat dressing, resulting in a fat content of about 2 percent. After avocado was added, the fat content jumped to 42 percent. The higher fat salad increased blood levels of lutein by 7 times and beta-carotene by an incredible 18 times!

In another study, subjects were fed salads using dressings with a different fat content. Salad with non-fat dressing resulted in negligible carotenoid absorption. Low-fat dressing improved nutrient absorption some, but full-fat dressing made a significant increase. The researchers were not only surprised by how adding fat improved nutrient absorption, but also how little is absorbed when no fat is included.

So if you want to get all the nutrients you can from tomatos, green beans, spinach, or any low-fat food, you should add a little fat. Adding a good source of fat in the diet is important in order to gain the most nutrition from our foods. Palm oil with all of its other health benefits makes an excellent choice.

Chapter 8

Palm Oil
Types and Uses

TYPES OF PALM OIL

There are several types of palm oil. All of them come from the same source. Red or virgin palm oil is becoming the most popular among individual consumers. White palm oil is preferred for commercial use. The basic difference between red and white palm oil is the degree of processing. In addition, there is fractionated palm oil. Fractionation is the separation of the different components or triglycerides. As you recall from Chapter 3, triglycerides are fat molecules composed of three fatty acids. Palm oil lends itself well to fractionation because it tends to separate naturally. Depending on the temperature, the different triglycerides form into liquid and solid fractions. The liquid portion can be poured off, leaving behind the more solid portion.

Each triglyceride has its own melting point. Saturated triglycerides have a higher melting point than monounsaturated triglycerides. And monounsaturated triglycerides have a higher melting point than polyunsaturated triglycerides. At controlled temperatures these triglycerides will separate out. When red palm oil is fractionated, the polyunsaturated triglycerides liquefy first, followed by the monounsaturated triglycerides. So the unsaturated portion of the oil can be separated, to some extent, from the saturated triglycerides. This process isn't pure, meaning the liquid portion isn't 100 percent unsaturated and the solid portion 100 percent saturated. What happens is that the liquid portion is enriched with unsaturated triglycerides and the solid portion is enriched with saturated triglycerides. These two fractions are called palm olein (liquid) and palm stearin (solid). The amount of unsaturated or saturated fatty acids can be controlled by the temperatures used in separation so that various degrees of palm olein and stearin can be produced.

The benefit of separating palm oil into olein and stearin fractions is that they can be used for different purposes. When a hard fat is needed for a certain recipe, such as croissants, palm oil stearin makes a perfect choice. When a liquid fat is needed, as in a salad dressing, palm oil olein is preferred. The most common types of palm oil sold in grocery stores are non-fractionated red palm oil, red palm oil olein, and white palm oil stearin (palm shortening). You may see both non-fractionated virgin palm oil and palm olein sold as "red palm oil." A way to tell the difference between the two is to observe them at room temperature: the virgin palm oil will be semi-solid while the palm olein will be mostly liquid.

The carotenoids which give palm oil its deep orange-red color have a melting point closer to the unsaturated portion. Therefore, palm olein has a richer amount of beta-carotene and other carotenoids. Consequently, palm stearin has a lesser amount and is whiter in color. When processed, it becomes pure white. This is palm shortening, which makes an excellent deep frying and bakery oil.

In nature the fatty acid content varies somewhat from one fruit to the next. The table on the opposite page shows an average fatty acid profile with mean ranges. Among chemists fatty acids are identified by a symbol CX:Y. The "C" represents the element carbon, and the first number (X) signifies the total number of carbons in the carbon chain of the fatty acid. The second number (Y) identifies whether it is a saturated fatty acid (0), monounsaturated fatty acid (1), or a polyunsaturated fatty acid (3 or more). For example, C16:0 represents the saturated fatty acid palmitic acid. The mean percent of palmitic acid in red palm oil is 44.2, with a range between 40.9 to 47.5 for samples tested in this table.

FATTY ACID COMPOSITION (wt. %)

Red Palm Oil

Fatty Acid	Mean	Range
Lauric C12:0	0.3	0.1 to 0.4
Myristic C14:0	1.2	1.0 to 1.4
Palmitic C16:0	44.2	40.9 to 47.5
Palmitoleic C16:1	0.3	0 to 0.6
Stearic C18:0	4.3	3.8 to 4.8
Oleic C18:1	38.8	36.4 to 41.2
Linoleic C18:2	10.4	9.2 to 11.6
Linolenic C18:3	0.3	0 to 0.5
Arachidic C20:0	0.4	0 to 0.8

Total Saturated 50
Total Unsaturated 50

Palm Olein

Fatty Acid	Mean	Range
Lauric C12:0	0.3	0.2 to 0.4
Myristic C14:0	1.1	0.9 to 1.2
Palmitic C16:0	40.6	38.2 to 42.9
Palmitoleic C16:1	0.2	0.1 to 0.3
Stearic C18:0	4.3	3.7 to 4.8
Oleic C18:1	41.9	39.8 to 43.9
Linoleic C18:2	11.6	10.4 to 12.7
Linolenic C18:3	0.4	0.1 to 0.6
Arachidic C20:0	0.4	0.2 to 0.6

Total Saturated 46
Total Unsaturated 54

Palm Stearin

Fatty Acid	Mean	Range
Lauric C12:0	0.2	0.1 to 0.3
Myristic C14:0	1.4	1.1 to 1.7
Palmitic C16:0	59.0	49.8 to 68.1
Palmitoleic C16:1	0.5	<0.05 to 0.1
Stearic C18:0	4.8	3.9 to 5.6
Oleic C18:1	27.4	20.4 to 34.4
Linoleic C18:2	7.0	5.0 to 8.9
Lenolenic C18:3	0.3	0.1 to 0.5
Arachidic C20:0	0.5	0.3 to 0.6

Total Saturated 65
Total Unsaturated 35

Source: *Pocketbook of Palm Oil Uses, Fifth Edition* September 2000, Malaysian Palm Oil Board. T.P. Pantzaris, editor Kuala Lumpur, Malaysia.

Melting Point

Oils generally do not have a sharp or precise melting point. Unlike water that melts at precisely 32 degrees F (0 C), oils change from a solid to a liquid over a range of temperatures. For this reason the melting point is determined by the temperate at which only 3-5 percent of solids are present. The melting point of virgin palm oil is 91-102 degrees F (33-39 C). Visually you can see both liquid and sold portions of the oil over a rather wide range of temperatures. At 50 degrees F (10 C) it has a mean solid fat content of 53.7 percent. So it appears mostly solid, yet is still relatively soft. At 104 degrees F (40 C) it is only 4.6 percent solid and looks completely liquid. At typical room temperatures of about 68 degrees F (20 C) palm oil has visible hard fat of 26 percent and may appear partially solid or liquid.

Solid Fat Content of Palm Oil:

10 C/50 F 53.7%
20 C/68 F 26.1%
30 C/86 F 10.5%
40 C/104 F 4.6%

Source: *Pocketbook of Palm Oil Uses, Fifth Edition* September 2000, Malaysian Palm Oil Board. T.P. Pantzaris, editor Kuala Lumpur, Malaysia.

PALM KERNEL OIL

The oil palm bears a fruit that produces two types of oils—palm oil and palm kernel oil. Palm oil comes from the pulp or flesh of the fruit while palm kernel oil comes from the seed or kernel. These two oils are very different from each other in both composition and effects on health.

Both the fruit and the seed contain a rich amount of oil, 49 percent in the fruit and 50 percent in the kernel. The fruit, which is larger and softer than the seed, yields a great deal more oil and, therefore, is of greater economic importance.

Both have a high saturated fat content with palm kernel oil having the higher of the two, as much as 82 percent compared to palm oil's 50

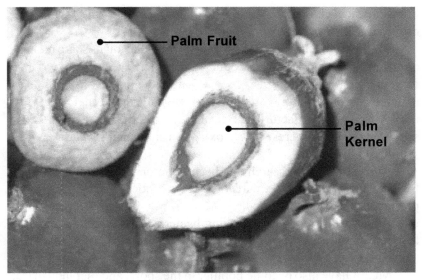

Palm Fruit

Palm Kernel

Palm oil comes from the fruit surrounding the seed (kernel). Palm kernel oil comes from the seed.

percent. Palm oil contains mainly palmitic (C16:0) and oleic (C18:1) fatty acids. Palm kernel oil contains primarily lauric acid (C12:0).

Both make stable cooking oils. Palm kernel oil has a much sharper, well-defined melting point of 76 degrees F (24 C), which makes it useful in commercial food industry, particularly in candy making where the melting point is crucial. Above this temperature it is completely liquid and, given enough time, below this temperature it is solid. Palm kernel oil is white in color when solid and colorless when liquid.

Palm kernel oil contains about an equal portion of tocopherols and tocotrienols, but the total vitamin E content is only a fraction of that of palm oil. It contains virtually no carotenes.

While palm kernel oil does not contain the abundance of phytonutrients that palm oil does, it is still a very healthy oil with many health benefits. Palm kernel oil is considered a lauric oil, meaning it is a rich source of lauric acid. The oil is composed predominately of medium-chain fatty acids—those with carbon chain numbers of 8, 10, and 12. About 56 percent of the fatty acids in palm kernel oil are classified as medium-chain fatty acids (MCFA). It's the MCFA that give palm kernel

137

oil its physical characteristics and health properties, both of which are different from those of palm oil.

The high content of lauric acid gives palm kernel oil its sharp melting point and solid composition at room temperature. These characteristics leave a clean, cool, non-greasy sensation on the palate, impossible to match using other natural oils. For this reason, palm kernel oil is very useful in food manufacturing. Because palm kernel oil is 82 percent saturated fat, it is very resistant to oxidation and rancidity and provides stability to foods.

A great deal of research has been done on the health aspects of MCFA. Perhaps the most remarkable characteristic is their antimicrobial properties. Research has shown that these fats protect us from infections by killing disease causing bacteria, viruses, and fungi. For this reason, MCFA are commonly used in foods, cosmetics, and medications.

MCFA have also become popular in the sports and diet industries. Unlike other fats, these fats do not contribute to the accumulation of body fat. They do just the opposite. They increase energy levels and stimulate metabolism, thus providing a boost of energy that accelerates

Fatty Acid Composition of Palm Kernel, Coconut, and Palm Oils

Fatty Acid	Palm Kernel	Coconut	Palm
Caproic C6:0	0.3	0.4	-
Caprylic C8:0	4.2	7.3	-
Capric C10:0	3.7	6.6	-
Lauric C12:0	48.7	47.8	0.2
Myristic C14:0	15.6	18.1	1.1
Palmitic C16:0	7.5	8.9	44.1
Stearic C18:0	1.8	2.7	4.4
Oleic C18:1	14.8	6.4	39.0
Linoleic C18:2	2.6	1.6	10.6
Others	0.1	0.1	0.75[a]

[a] C18:3, 0.37%; C20:0, 0.38%.

The above values are an average based on a number of samples analyzed.

the burning of calories. They are so effective that researchers are recommending them not only as a means for weight management, but also as a treatment for obesity. Sports enthusiasts like them because they improve energy levels and enhance performance. For this reason, many sports and fitness products on the market include them in their formulas. In foods and supplements, they are usually added as medium-chain triglycerides (MCT).

In addition to fighting off infections and enhancing energy, MCFA also support immune function, reduce chronic inflammation, and improve digestion. Research also shows they help protect against liver disease, kidney disease, cancer, and help to maintain balanced blood sugar levels.

In Africa where palm kernel oil has been used for thousands of years, it has a reputation as a healing oil. When people become sick, the remedy of choice among common folk is to drink a cup of palm kernel oil. Over the centuries they have learned that palm kernel oil is an effective remedy for many common illnesses.

Palm kernel oil is one of only two natural lauric oils. The other is coconut oil. The fatty acid profile of these two oils are remarkably similar. Consequently, the medicinal benefits of palm kernel oil and coconut oil are similar. For a more thorough description of the health benefits of medium-chain fatty acids, palm kernel oil, and coconut oil I recommend the books *The Coconut Oil Miracle* and *Coconut Cures*. See pages 165 and 166 for more information on these books.

PALM OIL IN FOOD PREPARATION

Fats enrich the flavor, taste, and texture of food and make it more palatable. Hard fats like lard, butter, and palm oil provide superior qualities over polyunsaturated vegetable oils in baking and frying. Taste, texture, appearance, and shelf life are all affected by the type of fat used. Unsaturated fats degrade quickly when heated and oxidize or become rancid, causing off flavors and producing harmful free radicals.

Fats are also used for greasing bread and baking trays and similar equipment. Unsaturated fats tend to polymerize and become gummy with repeated baking in the oven. If unsaturated fats are used in pan frying on the stove, polymerized vegetable oil can build up on the sides and underneath cookware and be overlooked during washing. This damaged oil residue builds up and appears as a hard amber-colored like varnish on the bottoms of pans. Once this varnish begins to build up it requires scouring or scrubbing to scrape it off the pan. This is why polyunsaturated oils have been useful in industrial use as paints and varnishes.

Hydrogenated vegetable oils act more like animal fats. They give baked and fried foods similar characteristics and do not polymerize like unsaturated fats. Hydrogenated fats were originally developed as a less expensive replacement for lard, beef fat, and butter in baked goods. As more people become aware of the dangers of trans fats, they are avoiding foods containing hydrogenated oils. In response, food manufacturers are seeking alternatives. Animal fats, while healthier than hydrogenated fats, are still viewed by many with suspicion. A perfect solution is palm oil. Food producers are recognizing the health benefits, and more and more products are appearing on grocery store shelves made with palm oil. Health enthusiasts are generally better educated about the nutritional and health aspects of foods. For this reason, palm oil has found a ready audience in health food stores.

Palm oil makes an excellent all purpose cooking oil. Because of its high saturated and low polyunsaturated fat content, it is ideal for cooking. It can be used in baking, sautéing, and deep frying. It produces a good mouth feel, retards oxidation and rancidity thus preserving flavor, helps to keep baked goods moist, and keeps crusts crispy and flaky. It is ideal for pastry dough. It makes excellent croissants and can used to make candy, cookies, cakes, breads, and even salad dressings.

Palm oil is easy to use. In recipes that call for margarine, shortening, vegetable oil, or any other type of fat, simply substitute in palm oil. Use the same proportions as called for in the recipe.

Palm oil can be used for all types of frying, including deep frying. Fried foods, and particularly deep fried foods, are considered taboo by many health conscious individuals because they are almost always cooked in hydrogenated oils. Oils used for deep frying often contain chemical additives, such as anti-foaming agents. Palm oil has a low foaming tendency so it doesn't need chemical additives. With palm oil you can enjoy French fries, scones, donuts, and other deep fried foods on occasion without worrying about them destroying your health.

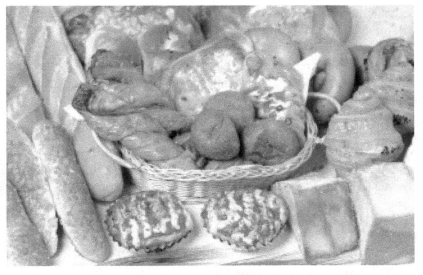

Palm oil can be used to make a variety of baked goods.

It's important that the fat used in deep frying be able to withstand high temperatures. The temperature at which an oil begins to smoke indicates how well it can tolerate heating and reheating. The higher the smoke point, the better. Typical frying temperature is about 360 degrees F (180 C). At this temperature unsaturated oils tend to either break down or be polymerized quite rapidly. This is why polyunsaturated vegetable oils are not recommended for frying. Palm oil, with a smoke point of 437 degrees F (225 C), well above normal frying temperatures, makes it an ideal frying oil. It is stable enough that it can be reused several times although you should skim or filter out debris from previous frying before reusing.

Unlike hydrogenated oils, palm oil does not leave a greasy feel in the mouth. This quality, in addition to the fact that it resists oxidation, has a low foaming tendency, and can withstand repeated use, makes palm oil ideal for commercial frying. In Western Europe and much of Southeast Asia, palm oil has become virtually the standard oil used in commercial kitchens.

Palm oil has a relatively high melting point. At room temperature it is semi-solid. On a cold day or when refrigerated, it hardens. On a hot day it may become completely liquid. In this aspect it is much like butter. When refrigerated butter is hard but, left out on a warm day, it will melt. There is no difference in the quality or health benefits of the oil when it is solid or liquid.

Since the oil resists oxidation, it does not need to be kept in the refrigerator. It will last for months stored in a cupboard at room temperature.

White or refined palm oil is generally used commercially. Red palm oil is the most popular among customers for home use. Because of its deep orange-red color, virgin palm oil tends to give foods an orange-yellow color. In most instances this is not a problem. Your stir fry vegetables will take on a faint orange color. Your fried chicken drippings will make a yellowish gravy. Curries look richer. Biscuits look buttery. However, in some foods you may not prefer the added color. For instance, a yellow colored angel food cake, loaf of bread, or mashed potatoes may take some getting used to. But it will make meals more colorful. For foods that you don't want colored, you, of course, can use another fat or use white palm oil or palm shortening (palm stearin).

Virgin palm oil has undergone minimal processing so it retains much of its natural aroma and flavor. The flavor of red palm oil can vary a great deal from brand to brand, depending on the processing methods used. Some brands may have a very strong, somewhat earthy flavor while others will be milder. Rancidity or poor processing procedures may intensify the earthy flavor. Cooking tempers the flavor somewhat so that even the strong flavored brands lose some of their bite. A good quality red palm oil has a mild, pleasant, savory flavor. When used in cooking, the oil can enhance the flavor of foods. It is especially good in sautés and curries. Many people use it as a condiment as they do butter to flavor foods. Add it to soup, vegetables, or pasta to enhance the flavor. Use it as the base for a salad dressing. You can even use it as a spread on bread or toast. I suggest you try several brands and use the ones that are the most appealing to you.

You can purchase red palm oil and trans fat free palm shortening at most good health foods stores as well as in a few grocery stores. Palm oil is often available in Brazilian, West African, and Asian markets. It is also sold on the Internet. As demand for healthy trans fat free oils increases, you will see various types of palm oil become more readily available.

DIETARY SUPPLEMENT

Palm oil can be used as a dietary supplement to provide a natural source of mixed vitamin E, mixed carotenoids, vitamin K, CoQ10, squalene, sterols, and other nutrients. The easiest way to take palm oil for its nutritional content is with foods. Use the oil in food preparation. You can also take the oil by the spoonful. One tablespoon (15 ml) of red palm oil provides equivalent of the adult US RDA of vitamin E and vitamin A (as provitamin A carotenes). For preschool aged children, 1 teaspoon (5 ml) satisfies the US RDA for these vitamins. Children ages 6-12 can take 2 teaspoons.

Palm oil is also available in gel capsules for those who want the benefits but can't handle taking the oil by the spoonful. The capsules are especially beneficial when you are away from home and can't use the oil in cooking.

Palm oil is non-toxic even in large amounts. It is a food, so it doesn't have any harmful side effects often associated with drugs. You could safely eat several tablespoons. The only potential drawback you might experience if you consume *large* amounts of red palm oil every single day is a slight yellowing of the skin. This is caused by the accumulation of carotenes in the skin. Carotenes, as you recall, are the pigments that give vegetables their orange color. This condition is not harmful in any way, and actually provides a great deal of protection to the skin from UV radiation and pollution. This condition is only temporary and will eventually go away if you stop eating the oil. Eating a couple of

Veterinarians Use Palm Oil

Because of its high nutrient content, red palm oil has become a popular dietary supplement recommended by veterinarians for birds, particularly parrots. It appears to provide birds with needed nutrients that brings about substantial improvement in health and appearance. Parrot owners report feathers becoming brighter and more colorful, feet becoming less flaky and scaly, beaks becoming smoother and taking on a healthy sheen. The birds gain relief from itching and scaling skin which keeps them from plucking their feathers. The end result is a happier, healthier pet.

Nutrient Content of Red Palm Oil

Approximate content of major nutrients in red palm oil per 1 tablespoon (14 g) serving.

Vitamin E

Alpha-tocopherol	2.26 mg
Alpha-tocotrienol	2.97 mg
Gamma-tocotrienol	4.68 mg
Delta-tocotrienol	1.28 mg
Total tocotrienols	8.94 mg
Total mixed vitamin E	11.20 mg

Carotenes

Alpha-carotene	2.59 mg
Beta-carotene	3.32 mg
Other carotenes	1.09 mg
Total mixed carotenes	7.00 mg

Other

CoQ10	600 mcg
Sterols	6 mg
Squalene	5 mg

tablespoons of red palm oil a day is not enough to color the skin. You would have to eat a large amount of the oil daily for an extended period of time for your skin to accumulate enough to become noticeable.

For those people who are not accustomed to eating much oil, you should be aware that, if you start adding 1 or more tablespoons of oil into your diet, it could loosen your bowels somewhat. This too is only a temporary condition. As your body adjusts to a larger amount of fat in the diet, you will no longer have this experience. If at first you experience loose bowels, all you need to do is cut back on the amount of oil you are using. As your body adjusts to the added fat, you can gradually increase the amount of oil you consume. Generally, if you replace the oils you normally use in your diet with palm oil, the amount of fat you are consuming remains the same and you will not notice any difference.

It is best to consume the oil with foods, either by cooking food in the oil or taking the oil along with meals. The oil improves the absorption of nutrients in the food. Also, oil digests more readily with food so there is less of a chance of experiencing abdominal discomfort or loose bowels.

TOPICAL USE OF PALM OIL

Palm oil is a natural antiaging, anticancer, antiwrinkle, moisturizing skin cream. It has a long history of use as a healing salve and topical ointment. As a folk remedy it is reported to relieve pain and speed the healing of wounds and injuries and dissolve tumorous growths. Many people even today swear of its healing powers. Judging from its chemical makeup, this makes sense. It contains a rich mixture of antioxidants as well as squalene, all of which strengthen and protect the skin. When palm oil is eaten or applied topically, these nutrients enrich the skin and underlying tissues.

Our skin is constantly being attacked by free radicals, the primary cause of wrinkles and sagging skin. Lipid peroxidation weakens connective tissues within the skin causing them to lose their elasticity. Facial wrinkles, therefore, are a sign of degeneration of the skin caused by free radicals. Wrinkles normally increase with age because of a lifetime exposure to oxidizing influences. Consuming palm oil or applying it on the skin can help to fight off the effects of free radicals and keep your skin looking younger.

UV light from the sun also generates free radicals that damage the skin and promotes premature aging as well as cancer. One of the most important therapeutic effects of palm oil is its photoprotective properties against UV radiation. Excessive exposure to sunlight can overwhelm the antioxidant defenses in our skin, causing sunburn and possibly leading to cancer. A way to provide protection to the skin would be to support the skin with antioxidants. Topical application of palm oil is an efficient way of enriching the skin with vitamin E and carotenes. The protection you get against damage caused by UV radiation using red palm oil applied on the skin is comparable to commercial SPF15 sunscreen.

Palm oil also helps improve skin health and enhances the skin's ability to heal. Palm oil shows promise as an aid in fighting skin cancer. Precancerous skin lesions are reported to disappear with the regular application of red palm oil. The skin becomes smoother, softer, and healthier. Injuries such as sunburn, burns, and cuts heal faster when palm oil is applied. The vitamin E and other nutrients are absorbed into the skin where they speed healing of injured tissue. The oil should be applied daily or several times a day. For quickest results put the oil on a bandage and keep it in constant contact with the skin until healed, changing the bandage as necessary. The idea is to keep the oil constantly in contact with the skin so that it can absorb as much of the oil's healing properties as possible.

Human skin testing has shown that red palm oil is safe on the skin even in high concentrations. A product that speeds healing, protects against cancer, protects the skin from the damaging effects of sunlight and pollution, helps prevent wrinkles, softens and moisturizes the skin and gives it a healthier appearance—without causing any harm—that's what you have with palm oil.

Though natural palm oil can be applied directly on the skin, there is one drawback: red palm oil stains the skin and your clothes a yellowish orange color. The color can be washed off your skin, but it's a much harder to remove from clothes. So you need to be careful.

One solution would be to consume the red palm oil and apply white palm oil on the skin. This way you gain all the benefits of the carotenes and other antioxidants in the red palm oil and the benefits of the tocotrienols in both the red and white palm oils. Palm kernel oil also has similar healing properties when applied topically. Palm kernel oil, which is colorless and won't stain the skin, actually is absorbed into the skin better than palm oil.

Note to Readers

Palm oil is helping many people enjoy a better level of health. I would like to know how palm oil is helping you. Please write and share your experiences with me. You can write to me in care of Piccadilly Books, Ltd., P.O. Box 25203, Colorado Springs, CO 80936, USA, or e-mail bruce@coconutresearchcenter.org. For more information about fats and oils ask for a free copy/ subscription to my *Healthy Ways Newsletter*. Subscriptions are only available via e-mail.

Chapter 9

Cooking with Palm Oil

There is no secret to using palm oil in cooking; simply replace other oils in your recipes with palm oil. Palm oil can replace both hard and liquid fats. The recipes in this chapter were patterned after traditional Malaysian, African, and Brazilian dishes that use palm oil. I have also added some recipes that are more familiar to American and European readers to demonstrate how palm oil can be used in a variety of ways.

MALAYSIAN FRIED CHICKEN
This is a uniquely flavored spicy fried chicken.

5 shallots, crushed or finely diced
4 cloves garlic, crushed or finely diced
½ teaspoon coriander powder
½ teaspoon cumin powder
½ teaspoon turmeric powder
1 teaspoon chili powder
1 teaspoon salt
1 teaspoon pepper
4-5 chicken drumsticks
Palm oil for frying

Combine all the seasonings to form a marinade. Cover chicken with marinade and let sit for at least 2 hours. Heat oil in pan over medium setting. Deep-fry the marinated chicken for about 5-6 minutes or until crispy and golden brown. Remove chicken and drain on paper towel. Serve hot.

MALAYSIAN STYLE CHICKEN SOUP

This is an interesting soup that will add spice to your life.

¼ cup red palm oil
1 cup onion, coarsely chopped
6 cloves garlic, finely chopped
¼ inch piece ginger, thinly sliced
2 cups chicken cut into bite-size pieces
1 tablespoon peanuts, finely chopped
1 teaspoon ground coriander
½ teaspoon chili powder
6 cups water
1 teaspoon salt
2 cups rice noodles, cooked
2 cups bean sprouts
2 eggs, hard boiled, sliced

Heat oil in a large pot. Sauté onions, garlic, and ginger until tender. Add chicken, peanuts, coriander, and chili powder and cook for about 3 minutes. Add water and salt and simmer for 45 minutes. Place an equal portion of noodles and bean sprouts into four bowls. Fill bowls with hot soup. Garnish with sliced egg and serve.

FRIED RICE WITH CHICKEN

In Malaysia this dish is called "nasi goreng dengan ayam." It is very similar to Chinese fried rice with which most of us are familiar. The recipe can be modified using different vegetables or with beef or shrimp in place of the chicken. The recipe below makes a great side dish; if you double the recipe it can be served as a main dish.

¼ *cup red palm oil*
¼ *cup onion, chopped*
4 garlic cloves, chopped
½ *stalk celery, chopped*
¼ *cup peas*
½ *cup chicken, cut-up into bite-size pieces*
1 egg, beaten
½ *teaspoon chili powder (optional)*
2½ cups cooked rice
Salt

Heat oil in skillet. Sauté vegetables until tender. Push vegetables to side of pan. Add chicken and egg to center of pan and cook until egg is done. Add chili powder and rice and mix with cooked vegetables. Chili powder can be omitted if you don't want a spicy dish. Continue to cook, stirring occasionally, for 4-5 minutes. Add salt to taste. Makes 3-4 servings.

SHRIMP CURRY
This recipe was inspired by dishes popular in Malaysia and Thailand.

1 pound noodles
2 tablespoons red palm oil
1 onion, chopped
4 garlic cloves, minced
2 carrots, sliced
1 red bell pepper, diced
1 tablespoon ground ginger
1 tablespoon flour
1 can (14 oz) coconut milk
1 tablespoon red curry paste
2 tablespoons fish sauce
1 pound shrimp, peeled and deveined
¼ *cup cilantro, finely chopped*

Prepare noodles according to package directions, drain, and set aside. Heat oil in skillet and sauté onion and garlic until tender. Add carrots, bell pepper, and ginger and sauté until vegetables are soft, about 6 minutes. Mix flour into coconut milk. Add coconut milk, curry paste, and fish sauce to skillet and cook until curry paste is well blended. Add shrimp, reduce heat and simmer 3 to 4 minutes or until shrimp are pink. Remove from heat and fold in noodles until well coated with sauce. Garnish with cilantro.

BEAN CAKES
These savory little cakes are sold on the streets in West Africa.

1 can (15 oz) black-eyed peas
½ small onion
2 small carrots
1 egg
Salt and pepper
¼ cup flour
½ cup palm oil

Drain all the liquid from the black-eyed peas. Chop onion and carrots and mix in food processor or blender with the black-eyed peas and egg. Stir in salt and pepper and flour. Heat oil in skillet over medium setting. Form mixture into several balls. Roll balls in flour and place in hot oil, flattening slightly so the cakes are about 2 inches in diameter and ¼-inch thick. Cook until crisp, turn and cook other side.

FRIED PLANTAINS
Plantains are cousins to the banana, but unlike bananas are not sweet. They are starchy. When cooked, they taste somewhat like a potato. Fried plantains resemble fried potatoes in taste and texture. This tasty snack is sold all over West Africa.

2 large plantains
2 cups palm oil
Salt

Plantains should be green and firm. Peal and cut the plantains crosswise into several ½-inch thick slices. Heat oil in a skillet. Place slices into the hot oil. The oil should be deep enough so that the slices float. Cook until the slices are crisp on the outside but soft inside (about 8-10 minutes). Remove from the oil and drain and add salt to taste.

MASHED YAMS WITH EGGS

This interesting recipe is from Ghana, Africa.

2 cups mashed yams
3 tablespoons grated onions
½ cup palm oil
1 ripe tomato, diced
6 hard-boiled eggs
Salt and pepper

Boil yams until tender then mash with a fork. In a saucepan, heat oil and fry onions until tender. Add tomatoes, remove from heat. Stir in mashed yolks from two hard-boiled eggs. Add mixture to mashed yams and stir until well blended and color is even. Put into a bowl and garnish with remaining eggs.

CHICKEN STEW WITH OKRA

This popular West African dish is usually served with a porridge-like side dish made from corn, sweet potato, plantain, or cassava. In this version you accompany it with rice.

¼ cup red palm oil
1 chicken, cut into serving-size pieces
1 medium onion, chopped
¼ cup water
2 tablespoons tomato paste
3 medium tomatoes, diced
4 garlic cloves, minced and mashed into a paste

1 teaspoon cayenne
2 teaspoons salt
½ cup smooth peanut butter
1¾ cups chicken broth
1 sweet potato
1 package (10 oz) frozen okra

Put oil in a large skillet and over moderate heat brown both sides of chicken, about 6 minutes. Transfer chicken to a heavy pot. In skillet, cook onions until tender. In a small bowl, mix water with tomato paste. Add tomato paste mixture, onions and oil, diced tomatoes, garlic paste, cayenne, and salt to chicken in pot. Stir peanut butter and 1 cup broth in a bowl until smooth. Add to chicken with remaining broth. Bring to a boil, reduce heat, and simmer, covered, stirring occasionally until chicken is tender, about 30 minutes. Peel sweet potato and cut into 1-inch pieces. Stir into stew along with okra and simmer, covered, until potato is tender but not mushy, about 10 minutes. Serve with rice. Makes 6 servings.

BEEF AND PLANTAIN STEW

Plantains are commonly eaten in West Africa. Although they resemble bananas, they are starchy rather than sweet and are eaten as vegetables. In this dish they are used much like we would use potatoes.

2 tablespoons red palm oil
1 large onion, chopped
1 large carrot, sliced
1 pound beef, cut into bite-size pieces
2 large tomatoes, chopped
2 cups water
1 cup peas
2 green plantains, sliced
1 can (14 oz) coconut milk
Salt and pepper to taste

Heat oil in large pot. Sauté onions and carrots until tender. Add beef, tomatoes, and water, bring to a boil, reduce heat, cover, and simmer for about 30 minutes. Add peas, plantains, coconut milk, salt, and pepper and continue to cook until plantains are tender, but not mushy.

FISH BENACHIN
In Gambia, Africa, "bena-chin" means "one-pot." All the ingredients are cooked together in a single pot. Benachin comes in many versions since just about anything on hand can be used to make this stew. You can also make it with beef or chicken.

¼ cup red palm oil
1 large onion, chopped
3 cloves garlic, chopped
1 green pepper, chopped
1-2 hot peppers, chopped
3 fish filets (any type)
1 yam or 2 cups pumpkin, cut into bite-size pieces
1 tomato, chopped
¼ head cabbage, chopped
¼ cup tomato paste
½ cup rice
3 cups water
Salt to taste

Heat oil in large pot, and sauté onions, garlic, green pepper, and hot pepper until tender. Add fish, yam, tomato, cabbage, rice, tomato paste, water, and salt. Bring to a boil, reduce heat, cover and simmer until rice is done, about 45 minutes.

BRAZILIAN SHRIMP STEW
Red palm oil is an essential ingredient in many ethnic dishes, including this Brazilian recipe, because it adds color and a distinctive flavor to foods.

1 ¼ pounds large shrimp, tail off
¼ teaspoon black pepper
1 ½ teaspoons salt
4 garlic cloves, minced
¼ cup fresh lemon juice
1 can (14 oz) diced tomatoes
3 tablespoons red palm oil
1 medium onion, chopped
1 green bell pepper, chopped
½ teaspoon cayenne
¼ cup coarsely chopped fresh cilantro
1 cup coconut milk
Cooked rice

Combine shrimp, black pepper, ½ teaspoon salt, garlic, and lemon juice and cover and chill for 20 minutes. Purée tomatoes with juice in a blender until smooth. Put oil in a skillet and over moderate heat cook onion and bell pepper until tender. Add cayenne, 1 tablespoon cilantro, and remaining teaspoon of salt, and cook for 1 minute, constantly stirring. Add tomato puree and simmer until mixture thickens, stirring as needed, about 15 minutes. Stir in coconut milk and bring to a boil, add shrimp mixture and cook for 5 minutes. Remove from heat. Stir in remaining cilantro and season with salt and pepper to taste. Serve with rice. Makes 6 servings.

PAN FRIED PORK CHOPS

This is a simple, but delicious recipe from Brazil. Pan drippings make an excellent sauce for vegetables. Suggested side dishes: green beans, broccoli, cauliflower, peas, potatoes, or yams.

¼ cup red palm oil
4 pork chops
1 medium onion, sliced
Salt and pepper to taste

Heat oil in skillet at medium setting. Put pork chops and onion slices in pan, cover, and cook. Turn pork chops and cook until browned. Add salt and pepper to taste. Remove pork chops. Pour onion slices and pan drippings over vegetable side dish.

BRAZILIAN RICE

Most Brazilians eat rice with beans for lunch or dinner every day. This is a typical rice recipe.

2 tablespoons red palm oil
1 small onion, chopped
1 clove garlic, chopped
1 medium tomato, chopped
1 cup rice
1½ cups water
1 teaspoon salt

Heat oil in skillet. Sauté onion and garlic until tender. Add rice and tomato and stir fry for about 2 minutes. Add water and salt, bring to a boil, reduce heat, and simmer for about 45 minutes or until rice is done.

FEIJOADA (Black Bean Stew)

Feijoada is one of the most popular dishes in Brazil. It is eaten in virtually every household throughout the year. It is made with black beans and lots of meat. Almost any type of meat can be used, but generally the dish includes sausage, pork, and beef and is usually served with rice. This is a simplified version.

3 tablespoons red palm oil
1 medium onion, chopped
6 cloves garlic, chopped
½ pound of link sausage, sliced
½ pound pork, cut into bite-size pieces
½ pound beef, cut into bite-size pieces
2 cans (15 oz ea) black beans
1 bay leaf
Salt and pepper to taste

Heat oil in skillet and sauté onions, garlic, and meats until vegetables are tender. Combine with the remaining ingredients in a large pot, add enough water to cover, bring to a boil, reduce heat, and simmer for 1 hour.

KALE AND ONIONS

This is a popular vegetable dish in Brazil and is often served with feijoada (black bean stew). Swiss chard can be substituted for the kale if you like.

2 tablespoons red palm oil
2 bunches fresh kale
1 small onion, chopped
1 clove garlic, chopped
Salt and pepper to taste

Remove the stems of the kale. Cut the leaves into thin strips. Heat the oil in a skillet and sauté onions and garlic until tender. Add kale, salt, and pepper and stir. Add a small amount of water, cover, and steam until kale is done.

POTATO WEDGES

These delicious baked potatoes taste like fat French fries.

4 potatoes
1-2 tablespoons red palm oil
Salt

Preheat oven to 400 degrees F (200 C). Peel each potato and slice lengthwise into about 8 wedges. Coat each wedge with a thin layer of oil. Place in a baking dish. Keep wedges separated so that they don't touch one another. Bake for 55 minutes or until outside is crispy and inside soft. Remove from oven and sprinkle with salt. You may also use seasoned salt or other seasons such as chili powder or onion powder.

SAUTED GREEN BEANS
This is a simple, tasty dish which highlights the flavor of the palm oil.

2 tablespoons red palm oil
4 cups fresh green beans
½ medium onion, sliced
1 cup mushrooms, sliced
Salt and pepper to taste

Heat oil in skillet. Sauté green beans and onions until vegetables are tender. Add mushrooms, salt, and pepper and cook uncovered, stirring occasionally, until mushrooms are done. Serve with pan drippings.

CUCUMBER TOMATO SALAD
This is a simple salad with a palm oil and vinegar dressing. The red palm oil gives the salad a distinctive flavor.

Salad
½ cucumber, peeled and sliced
1 large tomato, cut in wedges
1 scallion, chopped
½ green bell pepper, chopped

Dressing
2 tablespoons apple cider vinegar
1 tablespoon water
1 tablespoon red palm oil, melted
Dash of salt and pepper

Prepare vegetables and put into bowl. In a separate bowl, mix dressing ingredients. Pour dressing over vegetables.

PALM OIL MAYONNAISE
Red palm oil makes a nice mayonnaise with a distinctive dark yellow-orange color. The palm oil gives the mayonnaise a slight savory flavor

that can enhance the taste of sandwiches and salads. Mayonnaise can be stored in the refrigerator for several hours but must be used the day you make it. In the refrigerator the mayonnaise gradually hardens, just like palm oil does. When combined with other ingredients, such as in a potato salad, it will remain soft and creamy for several days.

2 egg yolks
2 tablespoons apple cider vinegar
½ tablespoon prepared mustard
⅛ teaspoon paprika
⅛ teaspoon salt
1¼ cup red palm oil, liquefied

Combine egg yolks, vinegar, mustard, paprika, and salt in a blender or food processor. Turn on the processor. While the machine is running, pour in melted (but not hot) palm oil very slowly in a fine steady stream. The secret to making good mayonnaise is to add the oil slowly. Mayonnaise will thicken as oil is added.

THOUSAND ISLAND DRESSING
Using palm oil mayonnaise, you can make a tasty Thousand Island salad dressing.

½ cup palm oil mayonnaise
2 tablespoons chili sauce or ketchup
¼ cup pickle relish
⅛ teaspoon paprika
Salt and pepper to taste

Mix all ingredients together in a bowl. Store in airtight container in refrigerator. Use on salads or as a dip.

SPICE COOKIES
Most cookie recipes normally use either butter or shortening. Palm shortening replaces these fats very well because it gives a similar texture and imparts no added flavor. Red palm oil will add flavor and works

158

best with recipes that are also flavorful. Here is an example that looks and tastes similar to a pumpkin cookie.

1 ¼ cups whole wheat flour
½ teaspoon baking powder
2 teaspoons cinnamon
½ teaspoon nutmeg
½ teaspoon salt
2 eggs
½ cup red palm oil
½ cup plus 2 tablespoons sugar
¼ cup plus 1 tablespoon brown sugar

Preheat oven to 375 degrees F (190 C). Mix flour with baking powder, cinnamon, nutmeg, and salt and set aside. Cream together eggs, oil, and sugars, then mix into dry ingredients. Drop well-rounded ½ teaspoonfuls on lightly greased baking sheets, spacing cookies 2-inches apart. Bake 10-12 minutes until lightly edged with brown. Transfer immediately to wire racks to cool. Makes about 2 dozen cookies.

BAKING POWDER BISCUITS

This is a traditional baking powder biscuit recipe. If you use red palm oil, these biscuits will take on a golden yellow color and a savory, almost butter-like flavor. For best results chill the palm oil so that it is hardened before mixing it into the flour.

2 cups sifted flour
1 teaspoon salt
1 tablespoon baking powder
⅓ cup chilled palm oil
¾ cup milk or coconut milk

Preheat oven to 450 degrees F (230 C). Sift flour with salt and baking powder into a bowel and cut in palm oil with a pastry blender until it achieves the texture of very coarse meal; make a well in center, pour in milk, and stir briskly with a fork just until dough holds together. Knead gently on a lightly floured board 7 or 8 times. Roll ½-inch thick and cut in rounds with a floured biscuit cutter; reroll and cut scraps. Place on ungreased baking sheet about 1-inch apart for crusty-sided biscuits, almost touching for soft. Bake for 12-15 minutes until slightly browned.

QUICK AND EASY BISCUITS
This is a simplified version of the above recipe. It produces a lighter, softer biscuit.

2 cups sifted flour
1 teaspoon salt
1 tablespoon baking powder
1 egg
⅓ cup palm oil, melted
¾ cup milk or coconut milk

Preheat oven to 450 degrees F (230 C). Sift flour with salt and baking powder into a bowl and set bowl aside. In a separate bowl blend together egg and liquid palm oil then stir in milk. Combine the liquid and dry ingredients and stir with a fork until dough holds together. Form dough into several balls about 2-inches in diameter. Place on ungreased baking sheet and flatten so that each biscuit is about ¾-inch thick. Bake for 12-15 minutes until slightly browned.

BRAN MUFFINS
These muffins are delicious. The red palm oil brings out the flavor.

1 cup water
1 tablespoon vanilla extract
⅓ cup honey
1 egg
¼ cup wheat bran
1 cup whole-wheat flour
2 teaspoons baking powder
¼ teaspoon salt
1 teaspoon cinnamon

½ teaspoon nutmeg
2 tablespoons melted red palm oil
½ cup chopped nuts

Combine water, vanilla, honey, egg, and bran in a bowl and let sit for about 10 minutes. The bran will absorb some of the moisture as it sits, which will improve the texture of the final product. In another bowl mix flour, baking powder, salt, cinnamon, and nutmeg. Preheat oven to 400 degrees F (200 C). Add melted palm oil (not hot) to the liquid ingredients, add the nuts, and mix together. Combine the wet and dry ingredients in one bowl and mix just until moist. Do not overmix or the muffins will not rise as well. Pour into greased muffin cups. Bake for 15 minutes. Makes 6 muffins.

CORN BREAD
This is a traditional recipe with a little tropical flair using palm oil and coconut milk. Can be made with either white or whole wheat flour. Produces a nice yellow corn bread.

1 cup sifted flour
1 cup sifted corn meal
1 tablespoon baking powder
¾ teaspoon salt
1 tablespoon honey
1 egg
1 cup milk or coconut milk
¼ cup red palm oil

Preheat oven to 400 degrees F (200 C). Sift flour, corn meal, baking powder, and salt into a bowl; beat egg with milk, honey, and oil just to blend. Make a well in dry ingredients, pour in egg mixture, and stir until well blended. Pour into a well-greased 8x8x2-inch baking pan and bake 20-25 minutes until bread pulls slightly from edges of pan, is lightly browned and springy to the touch. Cut in large squares and serve hot.

CROISSANTS

Nothing tastes better than fresh home-made croissants. This recipe, as with most pastries, works best with palm shortening. If you don't have palm shortening, you can use a half and half mixture of red palm oil and butter. The secret to making good croissants is to make sure that the dough and the shortening or palm oil/butter mixture is chilled.

¾ scalded milk
2 teaspoons sugar
1 teaspoon salt
¼ cup warm water
1 package active dry yeast
2¼-1½ cups sifted flour
½ cup palm shortening, chilled
1 egg yolk, lightly beaten with 1 tablespoon cold water (glaze)

Mix scalded milk, sugar, and salt and set aside to cool until lukewarm. Pour warm water into a warm mixing bowl, sprinkle in yeast, and stir to dissolve. Add cooled milk mixture, then mix in flour, a little at a time, to make a soft dough. Knead on a lightly floured board until elastic, about 5 minutes. Shape into a ball, place in a greased bowl, turning to grease

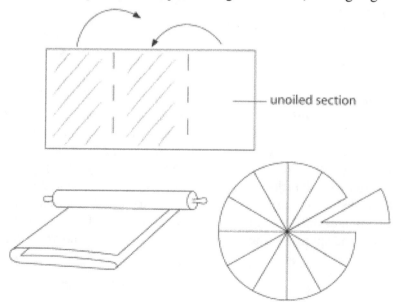

unoiled section

162

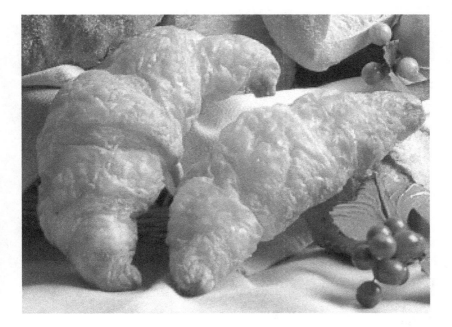

all over. Cover with cloth and let rise in a warm, draft-free place until doubled in bulk, about 1 hour. Punch down, wrap in wax paper, and chill 20 minutes. Meanwhile work palm shortening with your hands until pliable but still cold. Shortening or palm oil should not be melted. Roll dough on a lightly floured board into a rectangle about 12-inches x 16-inches. Spread half of the shortening over 2/3 of the dough and fold letter style, bring unoiled 1/3 in first. Pinch all edges to seal. Give dough 1/4 turn and roll quickly with short, even strokes into a 12-inch x 16-inch rectangle. Apply more shortening the same way, fold and roll again using remaining shortening. Roll and fold twice more (without adding any more shortening), then wrap and chill 2-3 hours or overnight. (Note: if kitchen is warm, chill dough as needed between rollings.) Halve dough, and keep 1 piece cold while shaping the other: roll into a 15-inch circle and cut like a pizza into 12 or 16 equal-size wedges. Starting from the wide side, roll up each piece loosely. Place 2-inches apart on ungreased baking sheets. Cover and let rise until almost doubled in size, about 1 hour. Toward end of rising, preheat oven to 375 degrees F (190 C). Brush rolls with glaze and bake 15-20 minutes until browned.

Appendix

Resources

USEFUL WEBSITES

American Palm Oil Council
www.americanpalmoil.com
This website is sponsored by the Malaysian Palm Oil Council. It contains a variety of interesting facts and articles regarding palm oil and its many uses.

Coconut Research Center
www.coconutresearchcenter.org
This website is sponsored by the Coconut Research Center. The Center is a nonprofit organization dedicated to educating the medical community and general public about the health aspects of coconut, palm, and other oils. This website contains numerous articles, current research, nutritional information, resources for educational materials and products, and includes an open discussion forum. A free subscription to the *Healthy Ways Newsletter* is available on request. Contact bruce@coconutresearchcenter.org.

Malaysian Palm Oil Council

www.mpopc.org.my

The Malaysian Palm Oil Council has sponsored a great deal of research and education on palm oil. It has been the world leader in promoting palm oil and educating the world on its many health benefits and industrial uses.

Palm Oil World

www.palmoilworld.org

This site contains a variety of interesting information about the benefits of palm oil.

Piccadilly Books, Ltd.

www.piccadillybooks.com

This website lists the best books and tapes currently available on the health aspects of tropical oils. Call or write and ask for a free catalog: Piccadilly Books, Ltd., P.O. Box 25203, Colorado Springs, CO 80936, USA, phone 719-550-9887, e-mail info@piccadillybooks.com.

The Price-Pottenger Nutrition Foundation

www.ppnf.org

This organization promotes research and education on nutrition, lifestyle, and health based on the works of Dr. Weston A. Price, Dr. Francis M. Pottenger, and others. They recognize the importance of healthy fats as an essential part of a wholesome diet.

Weston A. Price Foundation

www.westonaprice.org

This non-profit organization promotes the concept that health is strongly influenced by diet. Their website provides numerous articles on the importance of eating the right types of foods, including the right types of fat. They also provide resources for wholesome, natural foods.

BIBLIOGRAPHY

Coconut Cures: Preventing and Treating Common Health Problems with Coconut, Bruce Fife, 2005: Piccadilly Books, Ltd., Colorado Springs, CO.

The Coconut Oil Miracle, 4th Ed. Bruce Fife, 2004:Avery, New York, NY.

Eat Fat, Look Thin: A Safe and Natural Way to Lose Weight Permanently, 2nd Ed. Bruce Fife, 2005: Piccadilly Books, Ltd, Colorado Springs, CO.

Heart Frauds: Uncovering the Biggest Health Scam in History, Charles T. McGee, 2001: Piccadilly Books, Ltd, Colorado Springs, CO.

Nutrition and Physical Degeneration, 6th Ed., Weston A. Price, 1997: Keats Publishing, Los Angeles, CA.

The Oil Palm, 4th Ed., 2003, R.H.V. Corley and P. B. H. Tinker: Blackwell Publishing, Ltd., Oxford, UK.

Pocketbook of Palm Oil Uses, 5th Ed., T.P. Pantzaris: Malaysian Palm Oil Board, Kuala Lumpur, Malaysia.

The Trans Fat Dilemma and Natural Palm Oil, 2004, Gene A. Spiller: Pascoe Publishing, Rocklin, CA.

References

Chapter 2: The Trans Fat Attack

1. Raloff, J. Unusual fats lose heart-friendly image. *Science News* 1996;150:87.
2. Willett, W.C. Trans fatty acids and cardiovascular disease—epidemiological data. *Atherosclerosis* 2006;Suppl 7:5-8.

Chapter 3: The Facts on Fats

1. Prior, I. A. Cholesterol, coconuts, and diet on Polynesian atolls: a natural experiment: the Pukapuka and Tokelau island studies. *Am J Clin Nutr* 1981;34:1552-1561.
2. Mendis, S., et al. Cardiovascular risk factors in a Melanesian population apparently free from stroke and ischaemic heart disease: the Kitava study. *J Intern Med* 1994;236:331-340.
3. Mendis, S. Coronary heart disease and coronary risk profile in a primitive population. *Trop Geogr Med* 1991;43:199-202.
4. Ranvnskov, U. *The Cholesterol Myths.* Washington DC: New Trends Publishing, 2000.
5. Davis, G.P. and Park, E. *The Heart: The Living Pump.* New York: Torstar Books, 1983.
6. Mascioli, E.A., et al. Medium chain triglycerides and structured lipids as unique nonglucose energy sources in hyperalimentation. *Lipids* 1987;22:421-423.
7. Meade, C.J. and Mertin, J. Fatty acids and immunity. *Adv Lipid Res* 1978;16:127-165.
8. Carroll, K.K. and Khor, H.T. Effects of level and type of dietary fat on incidence of mammary tumors induced in female Sprague-Dawley rats by 7, 12-dimethylbenz(a)anthracene. *Lipids* 1971;6:415-420.
9. Whealan, J. Polyunsaturated fatty acids: signalling agents for intestinal cancer. *Nutr Today* 1997;32:213.
10. Cohen, L.A., et al. Dietary fat and mammary cancer. I. Promoting effect of different dietary fats on N-nitrosomethylurea-induced rat mammary tumorigenesis. *J Natl Cancer Inst* 1986;77:33-42.

11. Vinceti, M., et al. A population-based case-control study of diet and melanoma risk in northern Italy. *Public Health Nutr* 2005;8:1307-1314.

12. Ip, C., et al. Requirement of essential fatty acid for mammary tumorigenesis in the rat. *Cancer Res* 1985;45:1997-2001.

13. Kramer, J.K., et al. Reduction of myocardial necrosis in male albino rats by manipulation of dietary fatty acid levels. *Lipids* 1982;17:372-382.

14. Black, P.N. and Sharpe, S. Dietary fat and asthma: is there a connection? *Eur Respir J* 1997;10:6-12.

15. Harman, D., et al. Free radical theory of aging: effect of dietary fat on central nervous system function. *J Am Geriatr Soc* 1976;24:301-307.

16. Seddon, J.M., et al. Dietary fat and risk for advanced age-related macular degeneration. *Arch Ophthalmol* 2001;119:1191-1199.

17. Ouchi, M., et al. A novel relation of fatty acid with age-related macular degeneration. *Ophthalmologica* 2002;216:363-367.

18. Sheddon, J.M., et al. Progression of age-related macular degeneration: association with dietary fat, transunsaturated fat, nuts, and fish intake. *Arch Ophthalmol* 2003;121:1728-1737.

19. Packer, L. Protective role of vitamin E in biological systems. *Am J Clin Nutr* 1991;53:1050S-1055S.

20. Brigelius-Flohe, R. and Traber, M.G.. Vitamin E: function and metabolism. *FASEB J* 1999;13:1145-1155.

21. Rock, C.L., et al. Update on the biological characteristic of the antioxidant micronutrients: vitamin C, vitamin E and the carotenoids. *J Am Diet Assoc* 1996;96:633-699.

22. Aruoma, O.I. and Halliwell, B. eds. *Free Radicals and Food Additives*. London: Taylor and Francis, 1991.

23. Tewfik, I.H., et al. The effect of intermittent heating on some chemical parameters of refined oils used in Egypt. A public health nutrition concern. *Int J Food Sci Nutr* 1998;49:339-342.

24. Addis, P.B. and Wamer, G.J. *Free Radicals and Food Additives*. Aruoma, O.I. and Halliwell, B. eds. London:Taylor and Francis,1991.

25. Jurgens, G., et al. Immunostaining of human autopsy aortas with antibodies to modified apolipoprotein B and apoprotein(a) *Arterioscler Thromb* 1993;13:1689-1699.

26. Srivastava, S., et al. Identification of cardiac oxidoreductase(s) involved in the metabolism of the lipid peroxidation-derived aldehyde-4-hydroxynonenal. *Biochem J* 1998;329:469-475.

27. Nakamura, K., et al. Carvedilol decreases elevated oxidative stress in human failing myocardium. *Circulation* 2002;105:2867-2871.

28. Kritchevsky, D. and Tepper, S.A. Cholesterol vehicle in experimental atherosclerosis. 9. Comparison of heated corn oil and heated olive oil. *Journal of Atherosclerosis Research* 1967;7:647-651.

29. Pamplona, R., et al. Low fatty acid unsaturation: a mechanism for lowered lipoperoxidative modification of tissue proteins in mammalian species with long life spans. *J Gerontol A Biol Sci Med Sci* 2000;55:B286-B291.

30. Cha, Y.S. and Sachan, D.S. Oppostie effects of dietary saturated and unsaturated fatty acids on ethanol-pharmacokinetics, triglycerides and carnitines. *J Am Coll Nutr* 1994;13:338-343.

Chapter 4: Red Palm Oil

1. Khor, H.T. and Raajeswari, R. Red palm oil, vitamin A, and the antioxidant enzymes. In: *Micronutrients and Health: Molecular Biological Mechanisms.* Nesaretnam, K. and Packer, L (eds.) pp. 2990312. Champaign, IL:AOCS Press, 2001.

2.Packer, L. Protective role of vitamin E in biological systems *Am J Clin Nutr* 1991;53:1050S-1055S.

3. Elson, C.E. Tropical oils: nutritional and scientific issues. *Crit Rev Food Sci Nutr* 1992;31:79-102.

4. Kimmick, G..G.., et al. Vitamin E and breast cancer: a review *Nutr Cancer* 1997;27:109-117.

5. Gey, K.F., et al. Inverse correlation between plasma vitamin E and mortality from ischemic heart disease in cross-cultural epidemiology. *Am J Clin Nutr* 1991;53:326S-334S.

6. Passwater, R.A. *The Antioxidants.* New Canaan, CT: Keats Publishing, 1985.

7. Stampfer, M.J., et al. Vitamin E consumption and the risk of coronary disease in women. *N Eng J Med* 1993;328:1444-1449.

8. Rimm, E.B., et al. Vitamin E consumption and the risk of coronary heart disease in men. *N Eng J Med* 1993;328:1450-1456.

9. Lieberman, S. and Bruning, N. *The Real Vitamin and Mineral Book.* Garden City Park, NY:Avery Publishing Group, 1990.

10. Ethridge, E. Brain food. *Energy Times,* 1997;10:65.

11. Harman, D., et al. Free radical theory of aging: effect of dietary fat on central nervous system function. *J Am Geriatr Soc.* 1976;24:301-307.

12. Whitney, E.N., et al. *Understanding Normal and Clinical Nutrition, 3rd Ed.* St Paul, MN: West Publishing Company,1991.

13. Theriault, A., et al. Tocotrienol: a review of its therapeutic potential. *Clin Biochem* 1999;32:309-319.

14. Serbinova, E., et al. Free radical recycling and intermembrane mobility in the antioxidant properties of alpha-tocopherol and alpha-tocotrienol. *Free Radic Biol Med* 1991;10:263-275.

15. Nakamura, H., et al. Oral toxicity of a tocotrienol preparation in rats. *Food and Chemical Toxicology* 2001;39:799-805.

16. Mishima, K., et al. Vitamin E isoforms alpha-tocotrienol and gamma-tocopherol prevent cerebral infarction in mice. *Neurosci Lett* 2003;337:56-60.

17. Unchern, S., et al. The effects of vitamin E on platelet activity in beta-thalassaemia patients. *Br J Haematol* 2003;123:738-744.

18. Jiang, Q. and Ames, B.N. Gamma-tocopherol, but not alpha-tocopherol, decreases proinflammatory eicosanoids and inflammation damage in rats. *FASEB J* 2003;17:816-822.

19. Qureshi, A.A., et al. Dose-dependent suppression of serum cholesterol by tocotrienol-rich fraction (TRF25) of rice bran in hypercholesterolemic humans. *Atherosclerosis* 2002;161:199-207.

20. Tomeo, A.C., et al. Antioxidant effects of tocotrienols in patients with hyperlipidemia and carotid stenosis. *Lipids* 1995;30:1179-1183.

21. Malafa, M.P., et al. Vitamin E inhibits melanoma growth in mice. *Surgery* 2002;131:85-91.

22. Nesaretnam, K., et al. Effect of tocotrienols on the growth of a human breast cancer cell line in culture. *Lipids* 1995;30:1139-1143.

23. Wu, K., et al. Inhibitory effects of RRR-alpha-tocopheryl succinate on benozo(a)pyrene (B(a)P)-induced forestomach carcinogenesis in female mice. *World J Gastroenterol* 2001;7:60-65.

24. Musalmah, M, et al. Effect of vitamin E on plasma malondialdehyde, antioxidant enzyme levels and the rates of wound closures during wound healing in normal and diabetic rats. *Asia Pac J Clin Nutr* 2002;11 Suppl 7:S448-S451.

25. Nafeeza, M.I., et al. Comparative effects of a tocotrienol-rich fraction and tocopherol in aspirin-induced gastric lesions in rats. *Asia Pac J Clin Nutr* 2002;11:309-313.

26. Haas, A.L., et al. Vitamin E inhibits proliferation of human Tenon's capsule fibroblasts in vitro. *Ophthalmic Res* 1996;28:171-175.

27. Haas, A.L., et al. Inhibition of Tenon fibroblast proliferation. Comparison between Tocopherol and Mitomycin-C. *Invest Ophthalmol Vis Sci* 1996;37(suppl):877S.

28. Larrosa, J.M., et al. Alpha-tocopherol derivatives and wound healig in an experimental model of filtering surgery. *Ophthalmic Surg Lasers* 2000;31:131-135.

29. Pinilla, I., et al. Inhibitory effect of alpha tocopherol succinate on fibroblast wound healing. *Arch Soc Esp Oftalmol* 2000;75:383-388.

30. Sakamoto, T., et al. Vitamin E succinate inhibits proliferation and migration of retinal pigment epithelial cells in vitro: therapeutic implication for proliferative vitreoretinopathy. *Graefes Arch Clin Exp Ophthalmol* 1996;234:186-192.

31. Norazlina, M., et al. Tocotrienols are needed for normal bone calcification in growing female rats. *Asia Pac J Clin Nutr* 2002;11:194-199.

32. Machtey, I. and Ouaknine L. Tocopherol in osteoarthritis: a controlled pilot study. *J Am Geriatr Soc* 1978;26:328-330.

170

33. Blacnkenhorn, G.. Clinical efficacy of spondyvit (vitamin E) in activated arthoses. A multicenter, placebo-controlled, double-glind study. *Z Orthop* 1986;124:340-343.

34. Jacques, P.F., et al. Antioxidant status in persons with and without senile cataract. *Arch Ophthalmol* 1988;106:337-340.

35. Santos, M.S., et al. Beta-carotene-induced enhancement of natural killer cell activity in elderly men: an investigation of the role of cytokines. *Am J Clin Nutr* 1998;68:164-170.

36. Anonymous. Following the best science. *Life Extension* 1997;12:5-8.

37. Chew, B.P. and Park, J.S. Carotenoid action on the immune response. *J Nutr* 2004;134:257S-261S.

38. Myhre, A.M., et al. Water-miscible, emulsified, and solid forms of retinol supplements are more toxic than oil-based preparations. *Am J Clin Nutr* 2003;78:1152-1209.

39. Benade, A.J. A place for palm fruit oil to eliminate vitamin A deficiency. *Asia Pac J Clin Nutr* 2003;12:369-372.

40. Solomons, N.W. and Orozco, M. Alleviation of vitamin A deficiency with palm fruit and its products. *Asia Pac J Clin Nutr* 2003;12:373-384.

41. Sivan, Y.S., et al. Impact of vitamin A supplementation through different dosages of red palm oil and retinol palmitate on preschool children. *J Trop Pediatr* 2002;48:24-28.

42. Solomons, N.W. and Orozco, M. Alleviation of vitamin A deficiency with palm fruit and its products. *Asia Pac J Clin Nutr* 2003;12:373-384.

43. Hedren, E., et al. In vitro accessibility of carotenes from green leafy vegetables cooked with sunflower oil or red palm oil. *Int J Food Sci Nutr* 2002;53:445-453.

44. Solomons, N.W. and Orozco, M. Alleviation of vitamin A deficiency with palm fruit and its products. *Asia Pac J Clin Nutr* 2003;12:373-384.

45. Hedren, E., et al. In vitro accessibility of carotenes from green leafy vegetables cooked with sunflower oil or red palm oil. *Int J Food Sci Nutr* 2002;53:445-453.

46. Ali, et al. *Chest and Heart Journal* 2003;27:70-76. Cited in *Nutrition Briefs* July, 2004.

47. Canfield, L.M., et al. Red palm oil in the maternal diet increases provitamin A carotenoids in breastmilk and serum of the mother-infant dyad. *Eur J Nutr* 2001;40:30-38.

48. Zagre, N.M., et al. Red palm oil as a source of vitamin A for mothers and children: impact of a pilot project in Burkina Faso. *Public Health Nutr* 2003;6:733-742.

49. Strandberg, T.E., et al. Metabolic variables of cholesterol during squalene feeding in humans: comparison with cholestyramine treatment. *J Lipid Res* 1990;31:1637-1643.

171

50. Chan, P., et al. Effectiveness and safety of low-dose pravastatin and squalene, alone and in combination, in elderly patients with hypercholesterolemia. *J Clin Pharmacol* 1996;36:422-427.

51. Kohno, T., et al. Kinetic study of quenching reaction of singlet oxygen and scavenging reaction of free radical by squalene in n-butanol. *Biochim Biophys Acta* 1995;1256:52-56.

52. Storm, H.M., et al. Radioprotection of mice by dietary squalene. *Lipids* 1993;28:555-559.

53. Fliesler, S.J. and Keller, R.K. Isoprenoid metabolism in the vertebrate retina. *Int J Biochem Cell Biol* 1997;29:877-894.

54. Kamimura, H., et al. Enhanced elimination of theophylline, phenobarbital and strychnine from the bodies of rats and mice by squalane treatment. *J Pharmacobiodyn* 1992;15:215-221.

55. Richter, E., et al. Effects of dietary paraffin, squalane and sucrose polyester on residue disposition and elimination of hexachlorobenzene in rats. *Chem Biol Interact* 1982;40:335-344.

56. Richter, E. and Schafer, S.G. Effect of squalane on hexachlorobenzene (HCB) concentrations in tissues of mice. *J Environ Sci Health B* 1982;17:195-203.

57. Richter, E., et al. Stimulation of the faecal excretion of 2, 4, 5, 2', 4', 5'-hexachlorobiphenyl in rats by squalane. *Xenobiotica* 1983;13:337-343.

58. Smith, T.J., et al. Inhibition of 4-(methylnitrosamino)-1-(3-pyridyl)-1-butanone-induced lung tumorigenesis by dietary olive oil and squalene. *Carcinogenesis* 1998;19:703-706.

59. Fan, S.R., et al. Squalene inhibits sodium arsenite-induced sister chromatid exchanges and micronuclei in Chinese hamster ovary-K1 cells. *Mutat Res* 1996;368:165-169.

60. Murakoshi, M., et al. Inhibition by squalene of the tumor-promoting activity of 12-O-tetradecanoylphorbol-13-acetate in mouse-skin carcinogenesis. *Int J Cancer* 1992;52:950-952.

61. Rao, C.V., et al. Chemopreventive effect of squalene on colon cancer. *Carcinogenesis* 1998;19:287-290.

62. Littarru G.P., Lippa S., Oradei A., Fiorni R.M., Mazzanti L.Metabolic and diagnostic implications of blood CoQ10 levels. In: *Biomedical and Clinical Aspects of Coenzyme Q*, vol. 6 (1991) Folkers K., Yamagami T., and Littarru G. P. (eds)Elsevier, Amsterdam, pp 167-178.

63. Littarru G.P., Ho L., Folkers K. (1972) Deficiency of Coenzyme Q10 in human heart disease. Part I and II. In: *Internat. J. Vit. Nutr. Res.,* 42, n. 2, 291:42, n. 3:413.

64. Folkers K., Vadhanavikit S., Mortensen S.A. (1985) Biochemical rationale and myocardial tissue data on the effective therapy of cardiomyopathy with coenzyme Q10. In: *Proc. Natl. Acad. Sci., U.S.A.,* vol. 82(3), pp 901-904.

65. Mortensen S.A., Vadhanavikit S., Folkers K. (1984)Deficiency of coenzyme Q10 in myocardial failure. In: *Drugs Exptl. Clin. Res.* X(7) 497-502.

172

66. Kamikawa T., Kobayashi A., Yamashita T., Hayashi H., and Yamazaki N. (1985) Effects of coenzyme Q10 on exercise tolerance in chronic stable angina pectoris. In: *Am. J. Cardiol.*; 56:247-251.

67. Langsjoen Per.H., Vadhanavikit S., Folkers K. (1985) Response of patients in classes III and IV of cardiomyopathy to therapy in a blind and crossover trial with coenzyme Q10. In: *Proc. Natl. Acad. of Sci., U.S.A.,* vol. 82, pp 4240-4244.

68. Judy W.V., Hall J.H., Toth P.D., Folkers K. (1986) Double blind-double crossover study of coenzyme Q10 in heart failure. In: Folkers K., Yamamura Y. (eds) *Biomedical and clinical aspects of coenzyme Q,* vol. 5. Elsevier, Amsterdam, pp 315-323.

69. Schardt F., Welzel D., Schiess W., and Toda K. Effect of coenzyme Q10 on ischaemia-induced ST-segment depression: A double blind, placebo-controlled crossover study. In: *Biomedical and Clinical Aspects of Coenzyme Q,* vol. 6 (1991) Folkers K., Yamagami T., and Littarru G. P. (eds) Elsevier, Amsterdam, pp 385-403.

70. Rossi E., Lombardo A., Testa M., Lippa S., Oradei A., Littarru G.P., Lucente M. Coppola E., Manzoli U. Coenzyme Q10 in ischaemic cardiopathy. In: *Biomedical and Clinical Aspects of Coenzyme Q,* vol. 6 (1991) Folkers K., Yamagami T., and Littarru G. P. (eds) Elsevier, Amsterdam, pp 321-326.

71. Morisco C., Trimarco B., Condorelli M. Effect of coenzyme Q10 therapy in patients with congestive heart failure: A long-term multicenter randomized study. In: *Seventh International Symposium on Biomedical and Clinical Aspects of Coenzyme Q* Folkers K., Mortensen S.A., Littarru G.P., Yamagami T., and Lenaz G.. (eds) *The Clinical Investigator,* (1993) 71:S 34-S 136.

72. Langsjoen, P, et al. Treatment of essential hypertension with coenzyme Q10. *Mol Aspects Med* 1994;15 Suppl:S265-272.

73. Cortes E.P., Mohinder G.., Patel M., Mundia A., and Folkers K. Study of Administration of coenzyme Q10 to Adriamycin treated cancer patients. In: *Biomedical and Clinical Aspects of Coenzyme Q* (1977). Folkers K., Yamamura Y. (eds)Elsevier, Amsterdam, pp 267-273.

74. Folkers K., Langsjoen Per H., Willis R., Richardson P., Xia L., Ye C., Tamagawa H. (1990) Lovastatin decreases coenzyme Q levels in humans. *Proc. Natl. Acad Sci.* Vol. 87, pp.8931-8934.

75. Laaksonen, R., et al. Serum ubiquinone concentrations after short- and long-term treatment with HMG-CoA reductase inhibitors. *Eur J Clin Pharmacol* 1994;46:313-317.

76. Rusciani, L., et al. Low plasma coenzyme Q10 levels as an independent prognostic factor for melanoma progression. *J Am Acad Dermatol* 2006;54:234-241.

77. Lockwood, K., et al. Progress on therapy of breast cancer with vitamin Q10 and the regression of metastases. *Biochem Biophys Res Commun* 1995;212:172-177.

78. Lockwood, K., et al. Partial and complete regression of breast cancer in patients in relation to dosage of coenzyme Q10. *Biochem Biophys Res Commun* 1994;199:1504-1508.

79. Folkers, K., et al. The activities of coenzyme Q10 and vitamin B6 for immune responses. *Biochem Biophys Res Commun* 1993;193:88-92.

80. Hanioka, T., et al. Effect of topical application of coenzyme Q10 on adult periodontitis. *Mol Aspects Med* 1994;15 Suppl:S241-248.

81. Wilt, T.J., et al. Beta-sitosterol for the treatment of benign prostatic hyperplasia: a systematic review. *BJU Int* 1999;83:976-983.

82. Berges, R.R., et al. Randomised, placebo-controlled, double-blind clinical trial of beta-sitosterol in patients with benign prostatic hyperplasia. Beta-sitosterol Study Group. *Lancet* 1995;345:1529-1532.

83. Sundram, K., et al. Effect of dietary palm oils on mammary carcinogenesis in female rats induced by 7,12-Dimethylbenz(a)anthracene. *Cancer Res* 1989;49:1447-1451.

Chapater 5: Palm Oil and Cardiovascular Disease

1. Lees, A.M., et al. Plant sterols as cholesterol-lowering agents: clinical trials in patients with hypercholesterolemia and studies of sterol balance. *Atherosclerosis* 1977;28:325-338.

2. Jones, P.J., et al. Modulation of plasma lipid levels and cholesterol kinetics by phytosterol versus phytostanol esters. *J Lipid Res* 2000;41:697-705.

3. Pelletier, X., et al. A diet moderately enriched in phytosterols lowers plasma cholesterol concentrations in normocholesterolemic humans. *Ann Nutr Metab* 1995;39:291-295.

4. Fenton, C.V., et al. Dietary polyunsaturated fatty acids and composition of human aortic plaques. *Lancet* 1994;344:1195-1196.

5. Simopoulos, A.P., et al. The 1st Congress of the International Society for the Study of Fatty Acids and Lipids (ISSFAL): fatty acids and lipids from cell biology to human disease. *J Lipid Res* 1994;35:169-173.

6. Mensink, R.P. Effects of stearic acid on plasma lipid and lipoproteins in humans. *Lipids* 2005;40:1201-1205.

7. Hayes, K.C. Why the dietary fat issue is so complicated? *Proceedings of the International Society for the Study of Fatty Acids and Lipids (ISSFAL)* Winter, 1997.

8. Hayes, K.C. Saturated fats and blood lipids: new slant on an old story. *Can J Cardiol* 1995;11 Suppl G:39G-46G.

9. French, M.A., et al. Cholesterolaemic effect of palmitic acid in relation to other dietary fatty acids. *Asia Pac J Cliln Nutr* 2002;11 Suppl 7:S401-407.

10. van Jaarsveld, P.J., et al. Effect of palm olein oil in a moderate-fat diet on plasma lipoprotein profile and aortic atherosclerosis in non-human primates. *Asia Pac J Clin Nutr* 2002;11 Suppl 7:S424-432.

11. Zhang, J., et al. Nonhypercholesterolemic effects of a palm oil diet in Chinese adults. *J Nutr* 1997;127:509S-513S.

12. Chandrasekharan, N. Changing concepts in lipid nutrition in health and disease. *Med J Malaysia* 1999;54(3):408-427.

13. Qureshi, A.A., et al. Lowering of serum cholesterol in hypercholesterolemic humans by tocotrienols (palmvitee). *Am J Clin Nutr* 1991;53 Suppl:1021S-1026S.

14. Adams-Campbell, L.L., et al. Dietary assessment in Nigerian women: a pilot study. *Ethn Dis* 1993;3 Suppl:S62-626.

15. Ogunowo, P.O., et al. A clinical profile of patients with coronary artery disease in Nigeria. *Trop Georg Med* 1989;41:242-246.

16. Abengowe, C.U. Cardiovascular disease in Northen Nigeria. *Trop Geogr Med* 1979;31:553-560.

17. Kesteloot, H., et al. Serum lipid and apolipoprotein levels in a Nigerian population sample. *Atherosclerosis* 1989;78:33-38.

18. Collins, A.R., et al. Oxidative DNA damage measured in human lymphocytes: large differences between sexes and between countries, and correlations with heart disease mortality rates. *FASEB J* 1998;12:1397-400.

19. Gey, K., et al. Inverse correlation between plasma vitamin E and mortality from ischaemic heart disease in cross-cultural epidemiology. *Am J Clin Nutr* 1991;53:326S-3345.

20. Esterbauer, H., et al. Role of vitamin E in preventing the oxidation of low-density lipoprotein. *Am J Clin Nutr* 1991;3:314S-321S.

21. Esterbauer, H., et al. Vitamin E and other lipophilic antioxidants protect LDL against oxidation. *Fat Sci Technol* 1989;91:316-324.

22. Carew, T.E., et al. Antiatherogenic effect of probucol unrelated to its hypocholesterolemic effect: evidence that antioxidants in vivo can selectively inhibit low density lipoprotein degradation in macrophage-rich fatty streaks slowing the progression of atherosclerosis in the WHHL rabbit. *Proc Natl Acad Sci* 1987;84:7725-7729.

23. Singal, P.K. Role of free radicals in catecolamine-induced cardiomkyopathy. *Can J Physiol Pharmacol* 1982;60:1390-1397.

24. Tribble, D.L. AHA Science Advisory. Antioxidant consumption and the risk of coronary heart disease: emphasis on vitamin C, vitamin E, and beta-carotene: A statement for health care professionals from the American Heart Association. *Circulation* 1999;99:591-595.

25. Stampfer, M.J., et al. Vitamin E consumption and the risk of coronary disease in women. *N Engl J Med* 1993;328:1444-1449.

26. Rimm, E.B., et al. Vitamin E consumption and the risk of coronary heart disease in men. *N Engl J Med* 1993;328:1450-1456.

27. Stephens, N.G., et al. Randomized controlled trial of vitamin E in patients with coronary disease: Cambridge Heart Antioxidant Study (CHAOS). *Lancet* 1996;347:781-786.

28. Pereira, T.A., et al. Effects of dietary palm oil on serum lipid peroxidation, antithrombin III, plasma cyclilc AMP, and platelet aggregation. *Biochem Med Metab Biol* 1991;45(3):326-332.

29. Bayorh, M.A., et al. Effect of palm oil on blood pressure, endothelial function and oxidative stress. Food Technology & Nutrition Conference, 24-28 August 2003.

30. Tomeo, A.C., et al. Antioxidant effects of tocotrienols in patients with hyperlipidemia and carotid stenosis. *Lipids* 1995;30:1179-1183.

31. Qureshi, A.A., et al. Response of Hypercholesterolemic subjects to administration of tocotrienols. *Lipids* 1995;30:1171-1177.

32. Qureshi, A.A., et al. Lowering of serum cholesterol in hypercholesterolemic humans by tocotrienols (palmvitee). *Am J Clin Nutr* 1991;53(4)Suppl:1021S-1026S.

33. Tan, D.T.S., et al. Effect of a palm-oil-vitamin E concentrate on the serum and lipoprotein lipids in humans. *Am J Clin Nutr* 1991;53Suppl:1027S-1030S.

34. Kinosian, B., et al. Cholesterol and coronary heart disease: predicting risks by levels and ratios. *Ann Intern Med* 1994;121:641-647.

35. Qureshi, A.A., et al. Dietary tocotrienols reduce concentrations of plasma cholesterol, apolipoprotein B, thromboxane B2, and platelet factor 4 in pigs with inherited hyperlipidemias. *Am J Clin Nutr* 1991;53:1042S-1046S.

36. Sundram, K., et al. Replacement of dietary fat with palm oil: effect on human serum lipids, lipoproteins and Apo lipoproteins. *Br J Nutr* 1992;68:677-692.

37. Berg, K., et al. Lp(a) lipoprotein level predicts survival and major coronary events in the Scandinavian Simvastatin Survival Study. *Clin Genet* 1997;52:254-261.

38. Mensink, R.P., et al. Effect of dietary cis and trans fatty acids on serum lipoprotein(a) levels in humans. *J Lipid Res* 1992;33:1493-1501.

39. Jenkins, D.J., et al. Effect of a diet high in vegetables, fruit, and nuts on serum lipids. *Metabolism* 1997;46:530-537.

40. Theriault, A., et al Tocotrienol: a review of its therapeutic potential. *Clin Biochem* 1999;32:309-319.

41. Hornstra, G., et al. A palm oil-enriched diet lowers serum lipoprotein(a) in normocholesterolemic volunteers. *Atherosclerosis* 1991;90:91-93.

42. Ong, A.S. and Goh, S.H. Palm oil: a healthful and cost-effective dietary component. *Food Nutr Bull* 2002;23:11-22.

43. Wood, R., et al. Effect of palm oil, margarine, butter and sunflower oil on the serum lipids and lipoproteins of normocholesterolemic middle-aged men. *J Nutr Bio Chem* 1993;4:286-297.

44. Diaz, M.N., et al. Antioxidants and atherosclerotic heart disease. *N Engl J Med* 1997;337:408-416.

45. Unchern, S., et al. The effects of vitamin E on platelet activity in beta-thalassaemia patients. *Br J Haematol* 2003;123:738-744.

46. Ebong, P.E., et al. Influence of palm oil (Elaesis guineensis) on health. *Plant Foods Hum Nutr* 1999;53:209-222.

47. Ganafa, A.A., et al. Effect of palm oil on oxidative stress-induced hypertension in Sprague-Dawley rats. *Am J Hypertens* 2002;15:725-731.

48. Edem, D.O. Palm oil: biochemical, physiological, nutritional, hematological, and toxicological aspects: a review. *Plant Foods Hum Nutr* 2002;57:319-341.

49. Qureshi, A.A., et al. Dietary tocotrienols reduce concentrations of plasma cholesterol, apolipoprotein B, thromboxane B2, and platelet factor 4 in pigs with inherited hyperlipidemias. *Am J Clin Nutr* 1991;53:1042S-1046S.

50. Rand, M.L., et al. Effects of dietary palm oil on arterial thrombosis, platelet responses and platelet membrane fluidity in rat. *Lipids* 1988;23:1019-1023.

51. Pereira, T.A., et al. Effects dietary palm oil on serum lipid peroxidation, antithrombin III, plasma cyclic AMP, and platelet aggregation. *Biochem Med Metab Biol* 1990;45:326-332.

52. Ganafa, A.A., et al. Effect of palm oil on oxidative stress-induced hypertension in Sprague-Dawley rats. *Am J Hypertens* 2002;15:725-731.

53. Manning, R.D., et al. Oxidative stress and antioxidant treatment in hypertension and the associated renal damage. *American Journal of Nephrology* 2005;25:311-417.

54. Bayorh, M.A., et al. Effect of palm oil on blood pressure, endothelial function and oxidative stress. Food Technology & Nutrition Conference, 24-28 August 2003.

55. Ridker, P., et al. C-reactive protein and other markers of inflammation in the prediction of cardiovascular disease in women. *N Engl J Med* 2000;342:836-843.

56. Raloff, J., Vitamin E targets dangerous inflammation. *Science News* 2000;158:311.

57. O'Byrne, D., et al. Studies of LDL oxidation following a-, g-, d-tocotrienyl acetate supplementation of hypercholesteromic humans. *Free Radical Biology and Medicine* 2000;29:834.

58. Wang, X.L., et al. Cosupplementation with vitamin E and coenzyme Q10 reduces circulating markers of inflammation in baboons. *Am J Clin Nutr* 2004;80:649-655.

59. Engelberts, I., et al. The effect of replacement of dietary fat by palm oil on in vitro cytokine release. *Br J Nutr* 1993;69(1):159-167.

60. Esterhuyse, A.J., et al. Dietary red palm oil supplementation protects against the consequences of global ischemia in the isolated perfused rat heart. *Asia Pac J Clin Nutr* 2005;14:340-347.

61. Esterhuyse, A. J., et al. Dietary red palm oil improves reperfusion cardiac function in the isolated perfused rat heart of animals fed a high cholesterol diet. *Prostaglandins, Leukotrienes and Essential Fatty Acids* 2005;72:153-161.

62. Das, S. et al. Cardioprotection with palm tocotrienol: antioxidant activity of tocotrienol is linked with its ability to stabilize proteasomes. *Am J Physiol Heart Circ Physiol 2005*;289:H361-367.

63. Suarna, C., et al. Comparative antioxidant activity of tocotrienols and other natural lipid-soluble antioxidants in a homogeneous system, and in rat and human lipoproteins. *Biochem Biophys. Acta* 1993;1166:163-170.

64. Tomeo, A.C., et al. Antioxidant effects of tocotrienols in patients with hyperlipidemia and carotid stenosis. *Lipids* 1995;30:1179-1183.

65. Honstra, G., et al. Unexpected effect of dietary palm oil on atherothrombosis (rats) and atherosclerosis (rabbits). Comparison with other vegetable oils and fish oil. In: C. Galli and E. Fedelli (eds.), *Fat Production and Consumption: Technology and Nutritional Implications*, pp. 69-82. NATO-ASR Series A: Life Sciences. New York: Plenum Publishing Company, 1987.

Chapter 6: Fighting Cancer with Palm Oil

1. Steinmetz, KA. and Potter, J.D. Vegetables, fruits, and cancer prevention: a review. *J Am Diet Assoc* 1996;96:1027-1039.

2. Tan, B. Antitumor effects of palm carotenes and tocotrienols in HRS/J hairless female mice. *Nutr Res* 1992;12:S163-S173.

3. Nesaretnam, K., et al., Tocotrienol-rich fraction from palm oil and gene expression in human breast cancer cells. *Ann N Y Acad Sci* 2004;1031:143-157.

4. Nesaretnam, K., et al. Tocotrienols inhibit growth of ZR-75-1 breast cancer cells. *Int J Food Sco Nutr* 2000;51Suppl:S95-103.

5. McIntyre, B.S., et al. Antiproliferative and apoptotic effects of tocopherols and tocotrienols on preneoplastic and neoplastic mouse mammary epithelial cells. *Proc Soc Exp Biol Med* 2000;224:292-301.

6. Sylvester, P.W. and Shah, S.J. Mechanisms mediating the antiproliferative and apoptotic effects of vitamin E in mammary cancer cells. *Front Biosci* 2005;10:699-709.

7. Kalanithi, N., et al. Tocotrienol-rich fraction from palm oil affects gene expression in tumors resulting from MCF-7 cell inoculation in athymic mice. *Lipids* 2004;39:459-467.

8. Sylvester, P.W. and Shah, S. Antioxidants in dietary oils: their potential role in breast cancer prevention. *Mal J Nutr* 2002;8:1-11.

9. Sylvester, P.W., et al. Comparative effects of different animal and vegetable fats fed before and during carcinogen administration on mammary tumorigenesis, sexual maturation, and endocrine function in rats. *Cancer Res* 1986;46:757-762.

10. Nesaretnam, K., et al. Tocotrienols inhibit the growth of human breast cancer cells irrespective of estrogen receptor status *Lipids* 1998;33:461-469.

11. Kausar, H., et al. Palm oil alleviates 12-0-tetradecanoyl-phorbol-13-acetate-induced tumor promotion response in murine skin. *Cancer Lett* 2003;192:151-160.

178

12. Nishino, H., et al. Anticarcinogenesis activity of natural carotenes. *C R Seances Soc Biol Fil* 1989;183:85-89.

13. Malafa, M.P., et al. Vitamin E inhibits melanoma growth in mice. *Surgery* 2002;131:85-91.

14. Suda, D., et al. Inhibition of experimental oral carcinogenesis by topical beeta carotene. *Carcinogenesis* 1986;7:711-715.

15. Schwartz, J., et al. Beta carotene is associated with the regression of hamster buccal pouch carcinoma and the induction of tumor necrosis factor in macrophages. *Biochem Biophys Res Commun* 1986;136:1130-1135.

16. Zile, M.H., et al. Effect of moderate vitamin A supplementation and lack of dietary vitamin A on the development of mammary tumors in female rats treated with low carcinogenic dose levels of 7,12-dimethylbenz(a)anthracene. *Cancer Res* 1986;46:3495-3503.

17. Murakoshi, M., et al. Potent preventive action of alpha-carotene against carcinogenesis: spontaneous liver carcinogenesis and promoting stage of lung and skin carcinogenesis in mice are suppressed more effectively by alpha-carotene than by beta-carotene. *Cancer Res* 1992;52:6583-6587.

18. Har, C.H. and Keong, C.K. Effects of tocotrienols on cell viability and apoptosis in normal murine liver cells (BNL CL.2) and liver cancer cells (BNL 1ME A.7R.1), in vitro. *Asia Pac J Clin Nutr* 2005;14:374-380.

19. Wada, S., et al. Tumor suppressive effects of tocotrienol in vivo and in vitro. *Cancer Lett* 2005;229:181-191.

20. Yano, Y., et al. Induction of cytotoxicity in human lung adenocarcinoma cells by 6-0-carboxypropyl-alpha-tocotrienol, a redox-silent derivative of alpha-tocotrienol. *Int J Cancer* 2005;115(5):839-846.

21. Rahmat, A., et al. Long-term administration of tocotrienols and tumor-marker enzyme activities during hepatocarcinogenesis in rats. *Nutrition* 1993;9:229-232.

22. Nishino, H., et al. Anticarcinogenesis activity of natural carotenes. *C R Seances Soc Biol Fil* 1989;183:85-89.

23. Wu, K., et al. Inhibitory effects of RRR-alpha-tocopheryl succinate on benozo(a)pyrene (B(a)P)-induced forestomach carcinogenesis in feamale mice. *World J Gastroenterol* 2001;7:60-65.

24. Campbell, S., et al. Development of gamma (gamma)-tocopherol as a colorectal cancer chemopreventive agent. *Crit Rev Oncol Hematol* 2003;47(3):249-259.

25. Bostick, R.M., et al. Reduced risk of colon cancer with high intake of vitamin E: the Iowa Women's Health Study. *Cancer Res* 1993;53:4230-4237.

26. Agarwal, M.K., et al. Tocotrienol-rich fraction of palm oil activates p53, modulates Bax/Bcl2 ratio and induces apoptosis independent of cell cycle association. *Cell Cycle* 2004;3:205-211.

27. Srivastava, J.K. and Gupta, S. Tocotrienol-rich fraction of palm oil induces cell cycle arrest and apoptosis selectively in human prostate cancer cells. *Biochem Biophyss Res Commun* 2006;346:447-453.

28. Komiyama, K., et al. Studies on the biological activity of tocotrienols. *Chem Pharm Bull* 1989;37:1369-11371.

29. Clayman, C.B., editor. *The American Medical Association Encyclopedia of Medicine.* Random House: New York, 1989.

30. Kausar, H., et al. Palm oil alleviates 12-0-tetradecanoyl-phorbol-13-acetate-induced tumor promotion response in murine skin. *Cancer Lett* 2003;192:151-160.

31. Packer, L. and Landvik, S. Vitamin E: introduction to biochemistry and health benefits. *Ann NY Acad Sci* 1989;570:1-6.

32. Nesaretnam, K., et al. Tocotrienol-rich fraction from palm oil and gene expression in human breast cancer cells. *Ann N Y Acad Sci* 2004;1031:143-157.

33. Peto, R., et al. Can dietary beta-carotene materially reduce human cancer rates? *Nature* 1981;290:201-208.

34. Wolf, G. Is dietary beta-carotene an anticancer agent? *Nutr Rev* 1982;40:257-261.

35. Suda, D., et al. Inhibition of experimental oral carcinogenesis by topical beta-carotene. *Carcinogenesis* 1986;7:711-715.

36. Temple, N.J. and Basu, T.K. Protective effect of beta-carotene against colon tumors in mice. *J Natl Cancer Inst* 1987;78:1211-1214.

37. Zile, M.H., et al. Effect of moderate vitamin A supplementation and lack of dietary vitamin A on the development of mammary tumors in rats treated with low carcinogenic dose levels of 7,12-dimethylbenz(a)anthracene. *Cancer Res* 1986;46:3495-3503.

38. Malila, N., et al. Cancer incidence in a cohort of Finnish male smokers. *Eur J Cancer Prev* 2006;15:103-107.

39. Murakoshi, M., et al. Potent preventive action of alpha-carotene against carcinogenesis: spontaneous liver carcinogenesis and promoting stage of lung and skin carcinogenesis in mice are suppressed more effectively by alpha-carotene than by beta-carotene. *Cancer Res* 1992;52:6583-6587.

40. Nishino, H., et al. Anticarcinogenesis activity of natural carotenes. *C R Seances Soc Biol Fil* 1989;183:85-89.

41. Murakoshi, M., et al. Potent preventive action of alpha-carotene against carcinogenesis: spontaneous liver carcinogenesis and promoting stage of lung and skin carcinogenesis in mice are suppressed more effectively by alpha-carotene than by beta-carotene. *Cancer Res* 1992;52:6583-6587.

42. Ng, J.H., et al. Effect of retinoic acid and palm oil carotenoids on oestrone sulphatase and oestradiol-17beta hydroxysteroid dehydrogenase activities in MCF-7 and MDA-MB-231 breast cancer cell lines. *Int J Cancer* 2000;88:135-138.

43. Nesaretnam, K., et al. Effect of a carotene concentrate on the growth of human breast cancer cells and pS2 gene expression. *Toxicology* 2000;151:117-126.

44. Nesaretnam, K., et al. Effect of palm oil carotene on breast cancer tumorigenicity in nude mice. *Lipids* 2002;37:557-560.

45. Azuine, M A., et al. Antimutagenic and anticarcinogenic effects of carotenoids and dietary palm oil. *Nutr Cancer* 1992;17:287-295.

46. Nesaretnam, K., et al. Effect of toccotrienols on the growth of a human breast cancer cell line in culture. *Lipids* 1995;30(12):1139-43.

47. Wada, S., et al. Tumor suppressive effects of tocotrienol in vivo and in vitro. *Cancer Lett* 2005;229(2):181-191.

48. Nesaretnam, K., et al. Tocotrienols inhibit growth of ZR-75-1 mammary cancer cells. *Int J Food Sci Nutr* 2000;51:95-105.

49. Nesaretnam, K., et al. Effect of tocotrienols on the growth of a human breast cancer cell line in culture. *Lipids* 1995;30:1139-1143.

50. Carroll, K.K., et al. Anti-cancer properties of tocotrienols from palm oil, in *Nutrition, Lipids, Health, and Disease* (Ong, A.S.H., Niki, E., and Packer, L., eds.) pp.117-121, AOCS Press: Champaign, 1995.

51. Komiyama, K., et al. Studies on the biological activity of tocotrienols. *Chem Pharm Bull* 1989;37:1369-11371.

52. Goh, S.H., et al. Inhibition of tumour promotion by various palm oil tocotrienols. *Int J Cancer* 1994;57:529-531.

53. Rahmat, A., et al. Long-term administration of tocotrienols and tumor-marker enzyme activities during hepatocarcinogenesis in rats. *Nutrition* 1993;9:229-232.

54. Shah, S., et al. Role of caspase-8 activation in mediating vitamin E-induced apoptosis in murine mammary cancer cells. *Nutr Cancer* 2003;45:236-246.

55. Yano, Y., et al. Induction of cytotoxicity in human lung adenocarcinoma cells by 6-0-carboxypropyl-alpha-tocotrienol, a redox-silent derivative of alpha-tocotrienol. *Int J Cancer* 2005;115:839-846.

56. Gurhrie, N., et al. Palm oil tocotrienols and plant flavonoids act synergistically with each other and with Tamoxifen in inhibiting proliferation and growth of estrogen receptor-negative MDA-MB-435 and positive MCF-7 human breast cancer cells in culture. *Asia Pacific Journal of Clinical Nutrition* 1997;6:41-45.

57. Yu, W., et al. Induction of apoptosis in human breast cancer cells by tocopherols and tocotrienols. *Nutr Cancer* 1999;33:26-32.

58. McIntyre, B.S., et al. Antiproliferative and apoptotic effects of tocopherols and tocotrienols on normal mouse mammary epithelial cells *Lipids* 2000;35:171-180.

59. Sylvester, P.W., et al. Role of tocotrienols in the prevention of cardiovascular disease and breast cancer. *Curr Top Nutraceutical Res* 2003;1:121-136.

60. Shah, S., et al. Role of caspase-8 activation in mediating vitamin E-induced apoptosis in murine mammary cancer cells. *Nutr Cancer* 2003;45:236-246.

61. Agarwal, M.K., et al. Tocotrienol-rich fraction of palm oil activates p53, modulates Bax/Bcl2 ratio and induces apoptosis independent of cell cycle association. *Cell Cycle* 2004;3:205-211.

62. Nesaretnam, K., et al., Tocotrienol-rich fraction from palm oil and gene expression in human breast cancer cells. *Ann N Y Acad Sci* 2004;1031:143-157.

63. Sylvester, P.W. and Shah, S.J. Mechanisms mediating the antiproliferative and apoptotic effects of vitamin E in mammary cancer cells. *Front Biosci* 2005;10:699-709.

64. Shah, S., et al. Role of caspase-8 activation in mediating vitamin E-induced apoptosis in murine mammary cancer cells. *Nutr Cancer* 2003;45:236-246.

65. Sylvester, P.W., and Shah, S. Intracellular mechanisms mediating tocotrienol-induced apoptosis in neoplastic mammary epithelial cells. Food Technology & Nutrition Conference, 24-28 August 2003, International Palm Oil Congress.

66. Nesaretnam, K., et al. Tocotrienol-rich fraction from palm oil and gene expression in human breast cancer cells. *Ann N Y Acad Sci* 2004;1031:143-157.

67. Kalanithi, N., et al. Tocotrienol-rich fraction from palm oil affects gene expression in tumors resulting from MCF-7 cell inoculation in athymic mice. *Lipids* 2004;39:459-467.

68. Schwartz, J., et al. Beta carotene is associated with the regression of hamster buccal pouch carcinoma and the induction of tumor necrosis factor in macrophages. *Biochem Biophys Res Commun* 1986;136:1130-1135.

69. Ashfaq, M.K., et al. Vitamin E and beta-carotene affect natural killer cell function. *Int J Food Sci Nutr* 2000;51 Suppl:S13-20.

70. Nesaretnam, K., et al. Effect of palm oil carotene on breast cancer tumorigenicity in nude mince. *Lipids* 2002;37:557-560.

71. Sundram, K., et al. Effect of dietary palm oils on mammary carcinogenesis in female rats induced by 7,12-Dimethylbenz(a)anthracene. *Cancer Res* 1989;49:1447-1451.

72. Ip, C. Ability of dietary fat to overcome the resistance of mature female rates to 7,12-dimethylbenz(a)anthracene induced mammary tumorigenesis. *Cancer Res* 1985;40:2785-2789.

73. Sylvester, P.W., et al. Comparative effects of different animal and vegetable fats fed before and during carcinogen administration on mammary tumorigenesis, sexual maturation and endocrine functions in rats. *Cancer Res* 1986;46:757-762.

74. Kato, A., et al. Physiological effect of tocotrienol. *Yukagaku* 1985;34:375-376.

75. Fallon, S. and Enig, M.G. Diet and heart disease—not what you think. *Consumers' Research* 1996;79:15-19.

76. Chao, J.T., et al. Inhibitory effect of delta-tocotrienol, a HMG CoA reductase inhibitor, on monocyte-endothelial cell adhesion. *Nutr Sci Vitaminol* 2002;48:332-337.
77. Hayes, K.C., et al. Differences in the plasma transport and tissue concentrations of tocopherols and tocotrienols: observations in humans and hamsters. *Proc Soc Exp Biol Med* 1993;202:353-359.
78. Ohrvall, M., et al. Tocopherol concentrations in adipose tissue. Relationships of tocopherol concentrations and fatty acid composition in serum in a reference population of Swedish men and women. *Eur J Clin Nutr* 1994;48:212-218.
79. Sander, C.S., et al. Role of oxidative stress and the antioxidant network in cutaneous carcinogenesis. *Int J Dermatol* 2004;43:326-325.
80. Suda, D., et al. Inhibition of experimental oral carcinogenesis by topical beta carotene. *Carcinogenesis* 1986;7;711-715.
81. Schwartz, J., et al. Beta carotene is associated with the regression of hamster buccal pouch carcinoma and the induction of tumor necrosis factor in macrophages. *Biochem Biophys Res Commun* 1986;136:1130-1135.
82. Jens, J., et al. Ozone depletes tocopherols and tocotrienols topically applied to murine skin. *FEBS Letters* 1997;401:167-170.
83. Weber, C., et al. Efficacy of topically applied tocopherols and tocotrienols in protection of murine skin from oxidative damage induced by UV-irradiation. *Free Radic Biol Med* 1997;22:761-769.
84. Kausar, H., et al. Palm oil alleviates 12-0-tetradecanoyl-phorbol-13-acetate-induced tumor promotion response in murine skin. *Cancer Lett* 2003;192(2):151-160.

Chapter 7: A Health Tonic

1. Huang, Y, et al. Mechanism of free radicals on the molecular fluidity and chemical structure of the red cell membrane damage. *Clin Hemorheol Microcirc* 2000;23(2-4):287-290.
2. Ratnayake, W.M., et al. Vegetable oils high in phytosterols make erythrocytes less deformable and shorten the life span of stroke-prone spontaneously hypertensive rats. *J Nutr* 2000;130:1166-1178.
3. Brun, J.F. Hormones, metabolism and body composition as major determinants of blood theology: potential pathophysiological meaning. *Clin Hemorheol Microcirc* 2002;26:63-79.
4. Huang, Y., et al. Mechanism of free radicals on the molecular fluidity and chemical structure of the red cell membrane damage. *Clin Hemorheol Microcirc* 2000;23:2878-290.
5. Begum, A.N. and Terao, J. Protective effect of alpha-tocotrienol against free radical-induced impairment of erythrocyte deformability. *Biosci Biotechnol Biochem* 2002;66:398-403.

6. Senturk, U.K., et al. Effect of antioxidant vitamin treatment on the time course of hematological and hemorheological alterations after an exhausting exercise episode in human subjects. *J Appl Physiol* 2005;98:1272-1279.

7. Huang, Y., et al. Mechanism of free radicals on the molecular fluidity and chemical structure of the red cell membrane damage. *Clin Hemorheol Microcirc* 2000;23:2878-290.

8. Smith, J.A. Exercise, training and red blood cell turnover. *Sports Medicine* 1995;19:9-31.

9. Ratnayake, W.M., et al. Vegetable oils high in phytosterols make erythrocytes less deformable and shorten the life span of stroke-prone spontaneously hypertensive rats. *J Nutr* 2000;130:1166-1178.

10. Sevick, E.M. and Jain, R.K. Effect of red blood cell rigidity on tumor blood flow: increase in viscous resistance during hyperglycemia. *Cancer Res* 1991;51:2727-2730.

11. Ibanga, I.A., et al. Glycaemic control in type 2 diabetics and the mean corpuscular fragility. *Niger J Med* 2005;14:304-306.

12. Huang, Y., et al. Mechanism of free radicals on the molecular fluidity and chemical structure of the red cell membrane damage. *Clin Hemorheol Microcirc* 2000;23:2878-290.

13. Chiu, D.T. and Liu, T.Z. Free radical and oxidative damage in human blood cells. *J Biomed Sci* 1997;4:256-259.

14. Piagnerelli, M., et al. Red blood cell rheology in sepsis. *Intensive Care Med* 2003;29:1052-1061.

15. Langenfeld, J.E., et al. Red cell deformability is an early indicator of infection. *Surgery* 1991;110(2);398-403.

16. Nie, X., et al. Effects of morphine on rheological properties of rat red blood cells. *Clin Hemorheol Microcirc* 2000;22:189-195.

17. Korbut, R.A., et al. Endothelial secretogogues and deformability of erythrocytes. *J Physiol Pharmacol* 2002 53:655-665.

18. Bozzo, J., et al. Prohemorrhagic potential of dipyrone, ibuprofen, ketorolac, and aspirin: mechanisms associated with blood flow and erythrocyte deformability. *J Cardiovasc Pharmacol* 2002;38:183-190.

19. Shiraishi, K., et al. Impaired erythrocyte deformability and membrane fluidity in alcoholic liver disease: participation in disturbed hepatic microcirculation. *Alcohol* Suppl 1993;1A:59-64.

20. Smith, J.A. Exercise, training and red blood cell turnover. *Sports Medicine* 1995;19:9-31.

21. Bekyarova, G., et al. Reduced erythrocyte deformability related to activated lipid peroxidation during the early postburn period. *Burns* 1996;22:291-294.

22. Gelmini, G., et al. Evaluation of whole blood filterability with increasing age in healthy men and women. *Haematologica* 1989;74:15-18.

23. Begum, A.N. and Terao, J. Protective effect of alpha-tocotrienol against free radical-induced impairment of erythrocyte deformability. *Biosci Biotechnol Biochem* 2002;66:398-403.

24. Penco, M., et al. Modifications of whole blood filterability during acute myocardial infarction. *Clin Hemorheol Microcirc* 2000;22(2):153-159.

25. Solerte, S.B., et al. Hemorheological changes and overproduction of cytokines from immune cells in mild to moderate dementia of the Alzheimer's type: adverse effects on cerebromicrovascular system. *Neruobiol Aging* 2000;21:271-281.

26. Yao, J.K., et al. Red blood cell membrane dynamics in schizophrenia. III. Correlation of fatty acid abnormalities with clinical measures. *Schizophr Res* 1994;13:227-232.

27. Tomeo, A.C., et al. Antioxidant effects of tocotrienols in patients with hyperlipidemia and carotid stenosis. *Lipids* 1995;30:1179-1183.

28. Mishima, K., et al. Vitamin E isoforms alpha-tocotrienol and gamma-tocopherol prevent cerebral infarction in mice. *Neurosci Lett* 2003;337:56-60.

29. Kamat, J.P. and Devasagayam, T.P. Tocotrienols from palm oil as potent inhibitors of lipid peroxidation and protein oxidation in rat brain mitochondria. *Neurosci Lett* 1995;195:179-182.

30. Kabuto, H., et al. Melatonin inhibits iron-induced epileptic discharges in rats by suppressing peroxidation. *Epilepsia* 1998;39:237-243.

31. Beit-Yannai, E., et al. Cerebroprotective effect of stable nitroxide radicals in closed head injury in the rat. *Brain Res* 1996;717:22-28.

32. Keller, J.N., et al. Mitochondrial manganese superoxide dismutase prevents neural apoptosis and reduces ischemic brain injury: suppression of peroxynitrite production, lipid peroxidation, and mitochondrial dysfunction. *J Neurosci* 1998;18:687-697.

33. Kristian, T. and Siesjo, B.K. Calcium in ischemic cell death. *Stroke* 1998;29:705-718.

34. Borlongan, C.V., et al. Free radical damage and oxidative stress in Huntington's disease. *J Fla Med Assoc* 1996;83:335-341.

35. Smith, M.A., et al. Cytochemical demonstration of oxidative damage in Alzheimer disease by immunochemical enhancement of the carbonyl reaction with 2,4-dinitrophenylhydrazine. *H Histochem Cytochem* 1998;46:731-735.

36. Blaylock, R.L. *Excitotoxins: The Taste That Kills*. Health Press: Santa Fe, New Mexico, 1996.

37. Chandan, K. S., et al. Molecular basis of vitamin E action. *Journal of Biological Chemistry* 2000;275:13049-13055.

38. Khanna, S. et al. Molecular basis of vitamin E action: tocotrienol modulates 12-lipoxygenase, a key moderator of glutamate-induced neurodegeneration. *J Biol Chem* 2003;278:43508-43515.

39. Symeonidis, A., et al. Impairment of erythrocyte viscoelasticity is correlated with levels of glycosylated haemoglobin in diabetic patients. *Clin Lab Haematol* 2001;23:103-109.

40. Matkovics, B., et al. Pro-, antioxidant and filtration changes in the blood of type 1 diabetic patients. *Acta Physiol Hung* 1997-1998;85:99-106.

41. Chung, T.W., et al. Reducing lipid peroxidation stress of erythrocyte membrane by alpha-tocopherol nicotinate plays an important role in improving blood theological properties in type 2 diabetic patients with retinopathy. *Diabet Med* 1998;15:380-385.

42. Brown, C.D., et al. Association of reduced red blood cell deformability and diabetic nephropathy. *Kidney Int* 2005;67:295-300.

43. Nash, G..B., et al. Therapeutic aspects of white blood cell theology in severe ischaemia of the leg. *J Mal Vasc* 1991;16:32-34.

44. Harris, A.G.., et al. Leukocyte-capillary plugging and network resistance are increased in skeletal muscle of rats with streptozotocin-induced hyperglycemia. *Int J Microcirc Clin Exp* 1994;14:159-166.

45. Simpson, L.O. Intrinsic stiffening of red blood cells as the fundamental cause of diabetic nephropathy and microangiopathy: a new hypothesis. *Nephron* 1985;39:344-351.

46. Busijia, D.W., et al. Adverse effects of reactive oxygen species on vascular reactivity in insulin resistance. *Antioxid Redox Signal* 2006;8:1131-1140.

47. Haidara, M.A., et al. Role of oxidative stress in development of cardiovascular complications in diabetes mellitus. *Curr Vasc Pharmacol* 2006;4:215-227.

48. Senturk, U.K., et al. Effect of antioxidant vitamin treatment on the time course of hematological and hemorheological alterations after an exhausting exercise episode in human subjects. *J Appl Physiol* 2005;98:1272-1279.

49. Busiji, D.W., et al. Insulin resistance and associated dysfunction of resistance vessels and arterial hypertension. *Minerva Med* 2005;96:223-232.

50. Begum, A.N. and Terao, J. Protective effect of alpha-tocotrienol against free radical-induced impairment of erythrocyte deformability. *Biosci Biotechnol Biochem* 2002;66:398-403.

51. Brtko, J., et al. Nuclear all-trans retinoic acid receptors in liver of rats with diet-induced insulin resistance. *Ann N Y Acad Sci* 1997;827:480-484.

52. Sevick, E.M., Jain, R.K. Effect of red blood cell rigidity on tumor blood flow: increase in viscous resistance during hyperglycemia. *Cancer Res* 1991;51:2727-2730.

53. Storlien, L.H., et al. Fish oil prevents insulin resistance induced by high-fat feeding in rats. *Science* 1987;237:885-888.

54. Hunnicutt, J.W., et al. Saturated fatty acid-induced insulin resistance in rat adipocytes. *Diabetes* 1994;43:540-545.

55. Hollan, S. Membrane fluidity of blood cells. *Haematologia* 1996;27:109-127.

56. Nanji, A.A., et al. Dietary saturated fatty acids: a novel treatment for alcoholic liver disease. *Gastroenterology* 1995;109:617-620.

57. Purohit, V., et al. Role of fatty liver, dietary fatty acid supplements, and obesity in the progression of alcoholic liver disease: introduction and summary of the symposium. *Alcohol* 2004;34:3-8.

58. Nanji, A.A. and Tahan, S.R. Association between endothelial cell proliferation and pathologic changes in experimental alcoholic liver disease. *Toxicol Appl Pharmacol* 1996;140:101-107.

59. Mares, M., et al. Erythrocyte filterability and relative viscosity in liver cirrhosis and chronic hepatitis. *Clin Ter* 1989;129:243-259.

60. You, M., et al. Role of adiponectin in the protective action of dietary saturated fat against alcoholic fatty liver in mice. *Hepatology* 2005;42:568-577.

61. Ronis, M.J., et al. Dietary saturated fat reduces alcoholic hepatotoxicity in rats by altering fatty acid metabolism and membrane composition. *J Nutr* 2004;134:904-912.

62. Nanji, A.A., et al. Dietary saturated fatty acids reverse inflammatory and fibrotic changes in rat liver despite continued ethanol administration. *J Pharmacol Exp Ther* 2001;299:638-644.

63. Nanji, A.A., et al. Dietary saturated fatty acids; a novel treatment for alcoholic liver disease. *Gastroenterology* 1995;109:547-554.

64. Cha, Y.S. and Sachan, D.S. Oppostie effects of dietary saturated and unsaturated fatty acids on ethanol-pharmacokinetics, triglycerides and carnitines. *J Am Coll Nutr* 1994;13:338-343.

65. Pamplona, R., et al. Low fatty acid unsaturation: a mechanism for lowered lipoperoxidative modification of tissue proteins in mammalian species with long life spans. *J Gerontol A Biol Sci Med Sci* 2000;55:B286-B291.

66. Chang, C.C., et al. Asthma mortality; another opinion—is it a matter of life and…bread? *J Asthma* 1993;30:93-103.

67. Black, P.N. and Sharpe, S. Dietary fat and asthma: is there a connection? *Eur Respir J.* 1997;10:6-12.

68. Simchon, S., et al. Influence of reduced red cell deformability on regional blood flow. *Am J Physiol.* 1987;253:H898-903.

69. Todoriko, L.D. Changes in the morphofunctional state of the erythrocyte membranes in bronchial asthma in patients of different ages. *Lik Sprava* 1998 Mar-Apr;(2):51-54.

70. Schunemann, H.J., et al. Lung function in relation to intake of carotenoids and other antioxidant vitamins in a population-based study. *Am J Epidemiol* 2002;155:463-471.

71. Fife, B. *Eat Fat, Look Thin, 2nd Ed.* Colorado Springs. CO: Piccadilly Books, 2005.

Index